'With even a cursory glance at today's newspapers and news programmes one is led inescapably to the conclusion that the world is in a terrible mess, with violence, injustice, greed, slavery, drug addiction, crime and misery the normal living conditions for so many human beings. And yet all human beings want to be happy and indeed deserve to be happy. Countless numbers of people seek refuge in stimulants, depressants, drugs (legal and illegal), alcohol, coffee, sugar, dope, ecstasy et al. The phrase 'mind-altering substance' is often used by politicians as a 'catch-all' pejorative for the evils of the drug problem and conjures up images of mind control, of criminal conspiracies hell-bent on destroying 'civilisation as we know it'. But if there's one thing that needs to be altered in this troubled world it is the human mind, and if nature can offer us sound, safe, legal antidotes to the poisoning of the human spirit, then there can be no more important work in the 21st century than researching and exploring these resources.'

Sting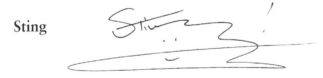

'*Natural Highs* gives you the goods on feeling fab. . . . I like this book a lot.'
Sarah Stacey, *YOU* magazine

'With science on its side, *Natural Highs* is the ideal handbook for helping everyone get a healthier happier life the natural way.'
Here's Health

'Patrick Holford puts the fun back into fitness . . . Holford is the new health cavalier, leading us clearly and intelligently to highs you don't have to pay for later.'
Jerome Burne, *Financial Times*

Patrick Holford, a trained psychologist, is the UK's leading nutritionist and one of the world's authorities on new approaches to health. In 1984 he founded The Institute for Optimum Nutrition, a charitable and educational trust for the furtherance of education and research in nutrition. It is now the largest training school in the UK for nutrition consultants and widely respected as a cutting edge organisation by professionals and media alike. He is the best-selling author of several books on nutrition.

Dr Hyla Cass, a graduate of the University of Toronto School of Medicine, is currently an Assistant Clinical Professor of Psychiatry at the UCLA School of Medicine. A prominent psychiatrist and expert on nutritional medicine, she is also a popular speaker and consultant on complementary medicine and psychiatry, women's health, stress reduction, and natural treatments for addictions, anxiety disorders and depression.

Other books by Patrick Holford

The Optimum Nutrition Bible
100% Health
The Optimum Nutrition Cookbook (with Judy Ridgway)
6 Weeks to Superhealth
Balancing Hormones Naturally (with Kate Neil)
Beat Stress and Fatigue
Boost Your Immune System (with Jennifer Meek)
Improve Your Digestion
Say No to Cancer
Say No to Heart Disease
Say No to Arthritis
The 30-Day Fatburner Diet
Supplements for Superhealth
The Little Book of Optimum Nutrition
Solve Your Skin Problems (with Natalie Savona)

Other books by Dr Hyla Cass

Kava: Nature's Answer to Stress, Anxiety and Insomnia (with Terence McNally)
St John's Wort: Nature's Blues Buster

NATURAL HIGHS

PATRICK HOLFORD & DR HYLA CASS

PIATKUS

Disclaimer

Natural Highs is intended solely for educational and information purposes and not as medical advice. Please consult a qualified medical or health professional if you have any questions about your health.

    While the nutritional supplements and herbs in the doses referred to in this book have been proven safe, neither the authors nor the publisher accept any liability should you choose to self-prescribe.

    All supplements should be kept out of the reach of infants and young children.

Copyright © 2001 by Patrick Holford and Hyla Cass

First published in 2001 by
Judy Piatkus (Publishers) Limited
5 Windmill Street
London W1T 2JA
www.piatkus.co.uk
e-mail: info@piatkus.co.uk

Reprinted 2001

The moral rights of the authors have been asserted

A catalogue record for this book is available from the British Library

ISBN 0 7499 2133 1

Edited by Barbara Kiser
Text design Sara Kidd
Illustrations by Jonathan Phillips

This book has been printed on paper manufactured
with respect for the environment using wood
from managed sustainable resources

Data capture and manipulation by Phoenix Photosetting, Chatham, Kent
Printed and bound in Great Britain by Mackays of Chatham, Kent

CONTENTS

ACKNOWLEDGEMENTS

This book would not have been possible without the help and support of many people.

I (Hyla) want to thank Jerry Cott, Ken Blum and Ann and Alexander Shulgin for their research input; Elaine Cass, Robert Zweben, my daughter, Alison, my mother Miriam Cass, and other family members and friends who advised and supported me; my patients who trusted me with their well-being; Terry McNally who helped me to write and re-write, and reminded me to take a break now and then; and Jim English, who has the gift of seeing my meaning and helping me communicate it more artfully. I want to thank the editorial team at Piatkus for being wonderfully patient, flexible and available, as well as talented in their craft; with a special thanks to Gill Bailey, who oversaw the entire project.

I (Patrick) would like to thank Alexander Shulgin, Dr Charles Grob, Oscar Ichazo, Dr Abram Hoffer, Dr Rick Strassman and many other people who have helped with guidance and research; and to Bebe Kohlap for taking care of things in my absences. A very special thanks goes to Natalie Savona for help with editing and to Rachel Winning and her team at Piatkus, especially Barbara Kiser, for their painstaking editing and design.

INTRODUCTION

IMAGINE A world where feeling happy, alert, energetic, relaxed and at one with the world is the norm. Where getting high is healthy and non-addictive. Sounds like science fiction?

It's all out there already. Or perhaps it's more accurate to say all *in* there, since, as we'll see, getting high is all about helping the brain get happy. We'll see how finding what does the job can be as easy as taking a swift trip to the supermarket, or scanning the shelves of your local health-food store.

Feel-good substances are already around in their hordes, of course. In an average week in Britain, we drink 1 billion cups of tea, 154 million coffees, 250 million sugared or caffeinated soft drinks and 120 million alcoholic drinks; smoke 1.5 billion cigarettes and consume 6 million kilograms of sugar and 2 million of chocolate. On top of this we take 2 million antidepressants, puff our way through 10 million joints and pop 1 million tabs of Ecstasy.

And do these work? Obviously they do, or they wouldn't be so popular. They boost energy, relieve anxiety, help us recover from a hard day's work. Cocaine can even help users feel 'better than good'. Except that the highs many of these substances give us can evaporate all too quickly, and leave us coping with a nasty aftermath.

Mood swings, depletion, exhaustion, and even addiction can result from all that popping, pouring and puffing. If you've quit, that's probably why. And if you haven't, it's probably why you're reading this book.

And it's all good news from here. We'll tell you about the natural alternatives – the healthy and legal ways to alter how you think and feel. You'll then be able to find your own perfect combination of diet, nutrients and techniques for staying naturally high. We'll show you:

▶ Hangover-free alternatives to relaxing with a beer.

▶ Nutrients that can help you reach heightened states of awareness or connection without the downsides of drugs.

▶ Foods that can replenish and restore a brain and body depleted by stress and excessive drug and alcohol use.

▶ Natural, non-addictive ways to get an energy kick like that from coffee, tea or tobacco.

▶ Natural alternatives to Prozac and Valium that work, with no side effects.

▶ How natural substances can help you escape from the prison of addiction.

At this point you may be questioning whether it is in fact natural to be high all the time! It certainly isn't the norm in our culture. In fact, there is evidence suggesting there may be evolutionary advantages to depression and anxiety. Being on edge, vigilant and watching for enemies and predators could have had greater survival value in the depths of prehistory than being blissed-out full time. Now, however, many people are on edge, anxious and/or depressed much of the time. If that sounds like you, the good news is that you can use mind-altering supplements and techniques to help break the patterns and open the way to a natural high.

Of course, 'natural' can mean a lot of things these days. Coffee, alcohol, nicotine, marijuana and even cocaine are all provided by Mother Nature, but they're not on the recommended list. By 'natural', then, we mean substances that are not only legal, but also good for you. They work with the body's design, not against it. They balance and add to health and energy rather than deplete it.

'High' is another loaded term. It can mean anything from the chemical variety to what we feel when we fall in love, see a magnificent sunset or ride a rollercoaster. Or the energy and exuberance most of us had as children.

It's Child's Play

Pass any schoolyard full of 5- or 6-year-olds, and what you notice is the energy, awareness and unselfconsciousness of this running, laughing, playing sea of kids. They engage with the world in a way that many of us have lost. It's rare to find a young child who is shy about singing, dancing and drawing in front of others, but how many of us would even contemplate doing the same?

Spontaneous and positive, kids are naturally high. They will go out of their way to enhance this too, by swinging on swings, or spinning in circles till they collapse. Even their crying and angry outbursts are a part of it, since expressing emotion is an essential part of this spontaneity. (Of course, not all childhoods are happy, and early trauma can certainly dampen this spontaneity.) As we approach adolescence, we become 'socialised' and lose some of this seemingly innate capacity for fun and pleasure.

Is it inevitable? Can't we stay energetic and open all the way into adulthood?

If we remind ourselves to stay present and aware, and keep trying new things, we have a fighting chance. Rote behaviour numbs us, and we forget to smell the flowers (sense awareness), appreciate our spouses (keeping our heart open) or are unable to accept a new way of doing something (mental flexibility). Thus, being more child-like – open, present and curious – is a key to sustaining mood, energy and connection. We have a whole section of exercises promoting sense awareness and mental flexibility, both attributes of childhood. And you can keep your energy levels up by following the diet and supplement suggestions.

Take Me Higher: Spirit and Transcendence

Another dimension of feeling high is the realm of transcendent or 'peak' experiences. In this state we feel a profound sense of unity or harmony, a deep connection with others, and a deeper awareness of life's purpose. It is the flash of inspiration that fuels great works of music, art and poetry, as well as scientific and spiritual breakthroughs. What's more, this shared human experience of connection with Nature, the Universe or God, while often difficult to describe in words, can actually be reflected on a brain scan!

Researchers have isolated a small portion of the emotional centre of the brain that is most active when we are having a spiritual experience. We may actually be hard-wired for this essential connection, with this area being a special receiving or connecting point. Scientists can even induce such an experience by electrically stimulating the area, labelled by Dr Michael Persinger at Laurentian University as 'the God module'.

Some people feel that the research is reducing the glory of spiritual experience by giving it an anatomical location. Others are excited by the concept that seems to prove the reality of this near-universal experience. Whatever your interpretation, though, if you have a functioning brain, it is very likely that you are able to get high.

While traditional cultures round the world have used psychoactive drugs to attain these peak states, we have other recommendations to help you get there. Besides specific combinations of herbs and nutrients, you will also discover methods to attain these states, such as meditation, movement, visualisation and special breathing techniques, in Part Three.

How We Work: The Mind-body Connection

Techniques like these depend upon the mind-body connection, with brain chemistry as the key link. The 'mind-body' interface is one of the hottest new areas of medical science and is helping us to understand for the first time just how it works and what we can do to improve our minds and moods.

The topic has fascinated both of us for over 20 years. As a psychiatrist (Hyla) and as a nutritionist specialising in mental health problems

(Patrick), we have worked with hundreds of clients who've had serious problems. By helping them modify their brain chemistry, we have both witnessed remarkable recoveries to robust mental health. Certain natural substances, we've found, really can help pull someone out of depression, recover balance in times of stress and promote an exhilarating sense of well-being.

We have also come across many people, especially those approaching middle age (it happens to the best of us!), who have an additional problem. They are less able to tolerate the use of alcohol, marijuana or other mind-altering substances that they once used freely. Others complain that the effect is diminished, that it 'just isn't what it used to be'. To their dismay, many have also noticed that their long-term substance use, even if it was only intermittent, has affected their mental abilities.

> Noel, a 45-year-old stock-broker and long-time pot-smoker, complained that 'Not only doesn't it work as well as it once did, but I feel so tired and foggy the next day, that the temporary high is just not worth it. My memory isn't as good as it used to be, either.'
>
> Fortunately, with the regular use of some prescribed supplements, Noel regained his mental faculties and energy. In fact, he claimed that 'I haven't felt this clear and energetic since I was in my twenties!' In the process he also lost his desire for smoking pot.

When you substitute 'pot' for alcohol, cigarettes, coffee or any other mind- and mood-altering substance, then you have an idea of the scope of the problem, and the effectiveness of our solution.

It sounds miraculous, and it is. As researchers unravel how natural mind-altering substances change our perceptions and moods, they've discovered an amazing thing: almost all these substances are similar to our own brain chemicals, and seem to work by mimicking, boosting or blocking their effects.

What this means, of course, is that we are all theoretically capable of producing our own natural highs, without even taking the substance.

How? The answer lies deep in our brains, with those chemical messengers of mind and emotion, the *neurotransmitters* (discussed in detail in Chapter 2).

As neurotransmitters are literally made from nutrients – amino acids, vitamins and minerals – we can formulate the perfect 'brain food' to improve how we feel and think. And certain nutritional supplements can create a state of high energy, increased focus and good mood. By taking these in the right combinations, well-being, connection and joie de vivre can become your normal state of mind.

Feeding your brain is vital. Just as important is remembering that chemistry works both ways: various substances can promote a natural high, *and* positive states of mind can raise the 'happy' brain chemicals. It's this crucial give and take that keeps us healthy and high.

How to Use This Book

Part One consists of three chapters, starting with the Natural High Questionnaire. The questionnaire will help you assess your own current needs, habits and patterns, and to develop your own strategy for shifting to natural highs.

We then introduce you to the basics of brain function. You will learn about neurotransmitters, the brain's 'communication chemicals' which are capable of stimulating and relaxing you, lifting your mood and sharpening your mind. You will find out why some substances knock your chemistry out of balance, while others are good for you. We then give you the **Natural High Basics**, a core regime of food and supplements that create the best internal environment for sustaining mood and energy. You will learn how to support your brain and body chemistry for maximum energy and balance.

Part Two is the heart of the book – five chapters that deal with the issues and substances that probably attracted you to this book in the first place: 'relaxants', 'stimulants', 'mood enhancers', 'mind and memory boosters' and 'connectors'. In each chapter, we follow a simple model in presenting the information:

▶ How you would prefer to feel, and how you might be feeling *now.*

▶ What goes on in your body and brain chemistry when you feel this way.

▶ The upsides and downsides of conventional substances that we use, such as alcohol and tranquillisers.

▶ The natural alternatives that can produce the desired result without the downsides. We'll learn why they work, the research on their benefits and how to use them.

▶ Finally, there's a straightforward action plan – clear and simple steps to achieve a natural high.

Part Three suggests other ways to achieve your natural high. You will see how breathing, meditation, exercise and sleep can raise mood and energy. We also look at positive thinking, sex and the life-enhancing uses of light, colour, music and aromatherapy.

Part Four offers top tips on natural ways to chill out, boost your energy, lift your mood, enhance your mind and get connected. There is also an A–Z listing of the substances you can take to achieve a natural high.

Guide to Abbreviations and Measures
1 gram (g) = 1000 milligrams (mg) = 1,000,000 micrograms (mcg)

Notes, Recommended Reading and Resources
In each part of the book we have numbered statements that link to research papers in the back of the book. These are there for those who wish to study this subject in depth. We also refer to more public oriented books and websites throughout the book, details of which can be found in Recommended Reading (page 302) and Resources (page 304) at the back of the book.

PART ONE

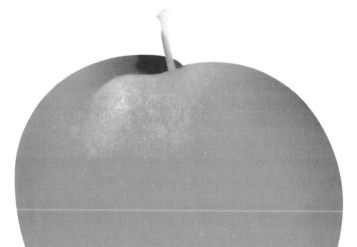

GETTING IN THE MOOD

HOW NATURALLY HIGH ARE YOU?

WE BELIEVE it is possible to be high – firing on all cylinders, inspired, enthusiastic, happy, calm and alert – most of the time. Our Natural High Programme promotes it by sustaining the right biochemical, physical and psychological conditions. There are four steps to being naturally high:

1. Achieve Optimum Brain Nutrition

When you improve your diet and take certain supplements, you can balance your blood sugar, which fuels brain and body, and supplies the building blocks for neurotransmitters, the brain's mood, mind and memory molecules. When you do this you find that you also break your dependency on substances that interfere with normal brain chemistry and deplete your energy.

2. Keep Yourself 'Fine-tuned' with Natural Highs

The reality of day-to-day life is that you can easily become stressed out or otherwise out of balance. You need to learn how to use natural substances to help bring yourself back into balance.

3. Think Positively

Chemistry isn't the whole story when it comes to natural highs. It's also about how we think. Ironically, we often have to work harder to achieve happiness, while fear and anxiety seem to come more easily. Fortunately, you can replace these negative patterns with a more positive and uplifting frame of mind.

4. Adopt a Naturally High Lifestyle

There are many ways to make yourself feel better – specific lifestyle changes in the form of physical, mental, emotional and spiritual exercises.

The **Natural High Programme** is designed to make it easy for you to make and maintain the step-by-step changes in your life that will allow you to be naturally and consistently high.

But before leaping headfirst into the mass of information that follows, check out the following Natural High Questionnaire, which will help you develop your personal natural high strategy.

The Natural High Questionnaire

Each of us is unique – an amalgam of genetic inheritance and a lifetime of experience. We may have inherited certain tendencies, for example to depression or anxiety. Together with what we learnt in childhood, and indulged in regularly as adults, these have programmed our body chemistry. We may have ended up, for instance, with a non-stop need for stimulation, or a seemingly built-in inability to relax.

The good news is none of this is set in stone. You *can* change.

The Natural High Questionnaire helps you find out what you need to work on. Each question relates to one or more of the following needs:

R for relaxation
S for stimulation
M for mood enhancement
I for IQ and memory boosting
C for connection, feeling part of everything, instead of apart

For any statement that is often true for you, highlight the entire box on the right-hand side. These contain the letters that denote the 'needs' revealed in that statement. When you've finished highlighting all the relevant boxes, add up your total score and interpret it, using the key on page 7.

For example:

STATEMENTS	R	S	M	I	C
I feel tired	R	S	M		
I have trouble getting going in the morning		S	M		
I am addicted to coffee, tea, cola or cigarettes		S			

The person who has completed these three statements has highlighted the first two and left the third statement clear. They have one R, three Ss and two Ms, which shows that overall they have a need for some relaxation and a higher need for stimulation and mood enhancement.

NATURAL HIGH QUESTIONNAIRE	R	S	M	I	C
I feel tired	R	S	M		
I have trouble getting going in the morning		S	M		
I need a cup of coffee, tea or cigarette to wake me up in the morning	R	S			
I abuse my body with a bad diet, drugs, overwork or lack of rest					C
I smoke or drink excessively (especially by others' standards)	R				
My energy seems to go up and down, and I often feel wiped out for no apparent reason		S			
I use sugar or caffeine (coffee, cola drinks) as a pick-me-up throughout the day		S			
Sometimes I feel foggy, fuzzy-headed		S		I	
I have difficulty concentrating	R	S		I	
I rely on a cup of coffee or tea or a cigarette to keep me thinking straight		S		I	
If I don't have caffeine or cigarettes I get a headache		S			
My moods seem to go up and down		S			
My mood swings are often relieved by food, especially sweets		S			
I think I'm addicted to coffee, caffeinated cola or cigarettes		S			
I find it hard to relax	R				C
I have a persistent feeling of fear or unease	R		M		
I am tense, irritable or impatient	R	S	M	I	C
I get a dry mouth and sweaty palms	R				

NATURAL HIGH QUESTIONNAIRE	R	S	M	I	C
I have little interest in sex	R				
I worry about little events of the day and am unable to shut my mind off	R				
I find it hard to relate to people	R				C
I am competitive and aggressive	R				
I eat quickly	R				
I have aching limbs or recurrent headaches	R				
I have crying spells or feel like crying			M		
My appetite is poor			M		
I feel unattractive and unlikeable			M		
It is an effort to do the things I used to			M		
I am restless and can't keep still	R		M		
My life feels pointless and I feel hopeless about the future			M		C
I get confused and find it difficult to make decisions			M	I	
I feel different, like the 'odd one out'					C
I often feel sad, angry or depressed			M		C
I don't have much enthusiasm for anything			M		C
I feel lonely much of the time and find it difficult to be alone					C
I am unclear about my spiritual values					C
I rarely have experiences of great joy or love					C
I rarely feel a connection with Nature					C
I feel disconnected from my local community					C
I rarely have peak or transcendent experiences where I feel at one with the world					C
My memory is deteriorating				I	
I sometimes forget the point I'm trying to make				I	
I sometimes meet someone I know quite well but can't remember their name				I	
I often find I can remember things from the past but forget what I did yesterday				I	
I sometimes go looking for something and forget what I'm looking for				I	
I find it harder to do calculations in my head				I	
I often experience mental tiredness				I	
I often misplace my keys				I	
I frequently repeat myself				I	
I have problems getting to sleep or sleeping through the night	R	S	M		

Count up the number of highlighted Rs, Ss, Ms, Is and Cs and make a note of the total for each one.

Total R = ☐ Total S = ☐ Total M = ☐ Total I = ☐ Total C = ☐

Now add up the totals for each letter to work out your overall score:

R + S + M + I + C = ☐   TOTAL

Interpreting the questionnaire

R for relaxation

8 or more: You are stressed out and need to make some major changes to your diet and lifestyle to avoid burnout. You must carefully follow the advice in Chapter 4.

4 to 7: You have a moderate imbalance, and will benefit from the advice in Chapter 4.

3 or less: You're in relatively good shape so far as relaxation is concerned.

S for stimulation

8 or more: Your 'get up and go' has got up and gone and you will need to make some major changes to your diet and lifestyle to get motivated. Carefully follow the advice in Chapter 5.

4 to 7: You have a moderate imbalance, and will benefit from the advice in Chapter 5.

3 or less: You're in relatively good shape so far as stimulation is concerned.

M for mood enhancement

8 or more: You need a mood boost, and should make some major changes to your diet and lifestyle to improve your mood, carefully following the advice in Chapter 6.

4 to 7: You have a moderate imbalance, and will benefit from the advice in Chapter 6.

3 or less: You're in relatively good shape as far as mood enhancement is concerned.

I for IQ and memory boost

8 or more: There's plenty of room for improvement in your memory and mental performance. You need to make some major changes to your diet and lifestyle to maximise your mental capabilities, and carefully follow the advice in Chapter 7.

4 to 7: You have a moderate imbalance, and will benefit from the advice in Chapter 7.

3 or less: You're in relatively good shape as far as IQ and memory are concerned.

C for connection

8 or more: You are very out of tune with others, and likely to feel and need to make some major changes to your diet and lifestyle to avoid burn-out. Carefully follow the advice in Chapter 8.

4 to 7: You have a moderate imbalance, and will benefit from the advice in Chapter 8.

3 or less: You're in relatively good shape.

Your Total Score

40 or more: You're seriously in need of a 'natural high' tune-up.

25 to 39: There is plenty of room for improvement in how you feel.

15 to 24: You have a moderate imbalance.

14 or less: You are already in good shape.

Whatever your score there's always some room for improvement. Once you've put our Natural High Programme into practice for 3 months, come back and check out how your scores have improved.

HOW YOUR BRAIN KEEPS YOU HIGH

THE BRAIN is incredible – a mere 1.3kg (3lb) in weight, and mainly composed of fat, it has the capacity to hold countless memories. It allows us to experience the delights of eating, the beauty of music, the ecstasy of love, the thrills of sex, and for some of us, the bliss of inner peace. It's also the abode of fear, anxiety and deep depression. Understanding how this phenomenon works will show you why coffee, say, works in the short term but not in the long term, and how natural highs get us up there to stay. We'll see why some substances knock your brain out of balance, and others make it hum.

The key to what's going on in our skull are special brain chemicals called neurotransmitters. They are the messengers of mind and mood.

Neurotransmitters: Getting the Message Across

You and I communicate with words. The brain communicates with neurotransmitters. These chemicals determine how you feel as they whizz round your brain and nervous system.

Trillions of nerve cells, called *neurons*, are scattered throughout the body but are most highly concentrated in the brain. Neurons connect to one another via branches called *dendrites* – 20,000 in all, linking together like interconnecting highways forming the 'road map' of our nervous system. Neurotransmitters, made from essential amino acids, are the couriers on these highways, delivering messages from one neuron to the next. To do this they have to cross small gaps between neurons called *synapses*. The 'sending' neuron produces the neurotransmitter, propelling it towards the 'receiving' neuron.

There's a slight complication though. The neurotransmitter is like a key that only fits into a certain lock on the receiving neuron called the *receptor site*. When these fit, the message is delivered – that is, the receptor is activated. An electrical signal then travels along the dendrites until it reaches the next synapse or road junction, where it triggers the release of more neurotransmitters.

Once a neurotransmitter has delivered its message, it's released from the receptor site and returns to the synapse. It might then be taken up once again into the neuron that sent it, where it can be used again, or it might be broken down and destroyed.

How you think and feel – your mood, alertness, level of relaxation and the state of your memory – are affected by the different levels of activity of different kinds of neurotransmitters. If there's a lot of one neurotransmitter you are likely to be happy; if there's a lack of another you are likely to feel unmotivated or tired.

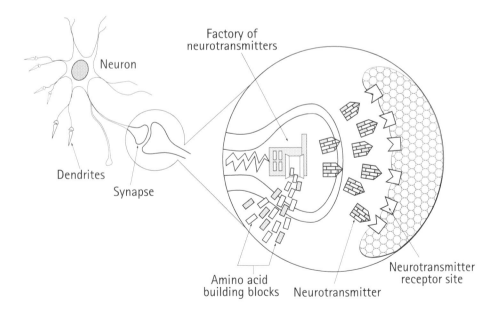

How neurotransmitters deliver messages from one neuron to another

Family tree of key neurotransmitters made from amino acids.

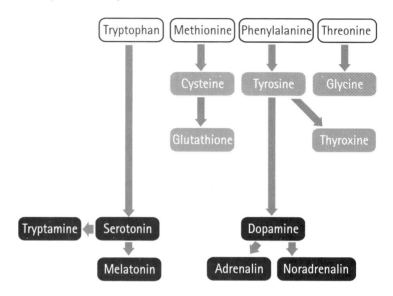

While there are hundreds of neurotransmitters, here are the main players:

▶ **GABA** is the 'cool' neurotransmitter, relaxing you and calming you down after stress.[1]

▶ **Adrenalin** is the 'motivator', stimulating you and helping you respond to stress.[2]

▶ **Dopamine** and **noradrenalin** are the 'feel-good' neurotransmitters, making you feel energised and in control.[3]

▶ **Endorphins** promote 'bliss', giving you a sense of euphoria.[4]

▶ **Serotonin** is the 'happy' neurotransmitter, improving your mood and banishing the blues.[5]

▶ **Acetylcholine** is the 'brainy' neurotransmitter, improving memory and mental alertness.[6]

(Endorphins and acetylcholine are not made from amino acids.)

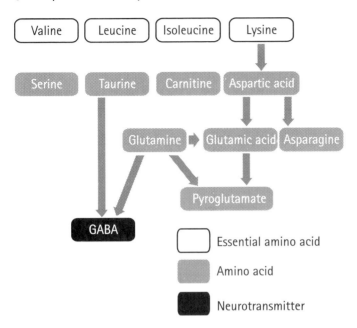

(See Notes, pages 291–3, for a more detailed description of what each of these neurotransmitters does and the symptoms associated with deficiencies of them.)

These are the big six – the key players in the orchestra of your brain and nervous system. The simple secret of being naturally high is that you have to find the right balance of substances and circumstances that get them really performing in perfect harmony.

The key to being naturally high is to know how to influence the balance of the brain's messengers. How can we possibly do this? Simple: remember, you are what you eat.

Neurotransmitters are made from amino acids, the building blocks of the protein you eat. There are eight essential amino acids (see above). From these eight we can make all the other amino acids our brain and body need, and from these we make neurotransmitters. In the figure above you can see how the neurotransmitter *serotonin* is made from the amino acid *tryptophan*. Serotonin is known to help improve your mood, so eating food rich in tryptophan, such as turkey, can improve your mood.

This was shown very clearly by an experiment carried out at Oxford University's Department of Psychiatry. Eight women were given a diet devoid of tryptophan. Within 8 hours, most of them started to feel more depressed. When tryptophan was added to their diet without their knowledge, their mood improved.[7] Tryptophan, then, is a natural high.

The popular antidepressant drugs, fluoxetine (Prozac) and sertraline (Zoloft) are called selective serotonin re-uptake inhibitors, or SSRIs. When we block the neurons' re-uptake of serotonin, there is more of the neurotransmitter available, which results in mood elevation. For more information see Chapter 6, page 111.

The Starbucks Effect

Every single mind-altering substance works by changing the balance of the neurotransmitters in your brain and nervous system. To better understand how, let's take a look at what happens when you drink a cup of coffee.

▶ Within minutes, you experience increased alertness and heightened focus.

▶ Your mood may improve, and your memory feel a bit sharper.

▶ You might also feel a bit jittery, and may soon have the urge to urinate (coffee is a diuretic).

▶ In an hour or two you might notice yourself feeling down, foggy and drowsy, and even irritable or cranky. You will probably start to crave another coffee at this point.

And this is what happens in your brain. The stimulant compounds in coffee – caffeine, theobromine and theophylline – cause the release of the neurotransmitter dopamine. Dopamine is then turned into adrenalin and noradrenalin. This trio of neurotransmitters leave you feeling motivated and stimulated.

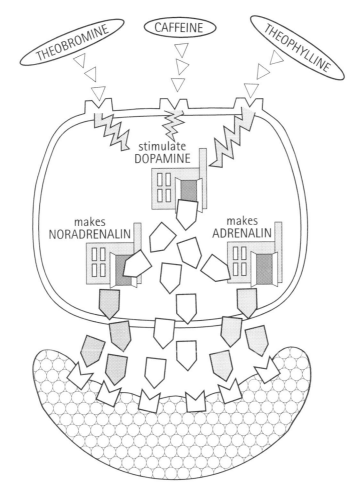

These neurotransmitters' signals raise blood sugar levels

How coffee gives you a kick

At the same time, adrenalin causes glucose, or blood sugar, to be released into your system, stimulating both mind and body, much as a hit of sugar, say from a doughnut, energises your body. Adrenalin also acts as a diuretic and makes you want to urinate.

But the effects don't end there. In an hour or two, it's as if you never had that coffee – and you're likely to want another one. Unfortunately, the next cup, or the cup after that, is unlikely to provide the same kick. Frequent consumption results in a diminished response known as 'tolerance'. So in time, you may graduate from a regular coffee to a 'grande', or a stronger brew.

Now you're addicted. If you don't get your morning fix of coffee you feel lousy, perhaps even headachy. This is due to 'withdrawal', the negative symptoms that appear when a substance is stopped and disappear when it is reinstated. Soon, the consumer is in the grip of a compulsion, and is addicted to the substance. Most of what we use to get high, from coffee to cocaine and cigarettes to alcohol, fall into this category. You get less and less benefit as you become more and more addicted. It's a bad deal.

Why Doesn't it Last? The Brain's Ups and Downs

Why do you need more and more caffeine, nicotine or alcohol to get the same effect? Remember the kick from your first cigarette? Have you ever wondered why you don't experience that any more?

The brain has a set of negative feedback mechanisms whose goal is to prevent us from being too stimulated for too long. When we boost our feel-good neurotransmitters, as we do with a cup of coffee, the dopamine released causes a feeling of well-being. However, in response, the receptors gradually shut down, deflating our high.

A key concept in the body and brain, as in all of nature, is balance. Much as a thermostat keeps our home at a desired temperature, our body has ways of maintaining a state of equilibrium. It doesn't want us to be too high for too long!

So, in response to an increase in the amount of neurotransmitter available, for example dopamine from drinking coffee, there is a 'downregulation' of the receptor sites. This means that some receptor sites shut down, making the neuron less responsive. Consequently you need more of the stimulant – caffeine, nicotine, cocaine, whatever – to release neurotransmitters into the synapses and get the message across. It's as if to block out the yelling of the neurotransmitters, the receptors put on

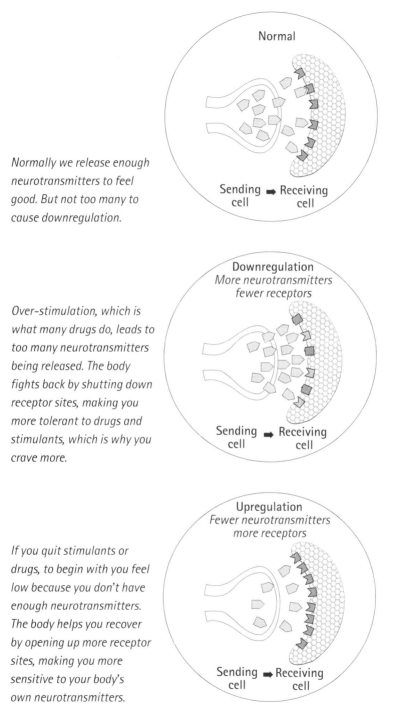

Normally we release enough neurotransmitters to feel good. But not too many to cause downregulation.

Normal

Sending ➡ Receiving
cell   cell

Over-stimulation, which is what many drugs do, leads to too many neurotransmitters being released. The body fights back by shutting down receptor sites, making you more tolerant to drugs and stimulants, which is why you crave more.

Downregulation
More neurotransmitters fewer receptors

Sending ➡ Receiving
cell   cell

If you quit stimulants or drugs, to begin with you feel low because you don't have enough neurotransmitters. The body helps you recover by opening up more receptor sites, making you more sensitive to your body's own neurotransmitters.

Upregulation
Fewer neurotransmitters more receptors

Sending ➡ Receiving
cell   cell

earplugs leaving the neurotransmitters no alternative but to yell even louder.

The body's self-regulation process, then, makes it impossible for us to gain any long-term benefit from the use of stimulants. Herein lies the rub.

The net result of addiction is that once the initial effect has worn off, the body's normal production of dopamine – its usual 'talking voice' – just isn't loud enough to get the now somewhat deaf neighbouring cells excited. As a consequence, you feel tired, lacking in motivation and in need of another hit of stimulant. And as time goes on you need more and more. No longer will that regular cup of coffee (around 100mg of caffeine) give you the kick-start you need. You need a large 'special' coffee (around 400mg), perhaps with a cigarette thrown in, or even a mochaccino (chocolate plus coffee, two different sources of caffeine).

Of course, the more you have and the more often you have it, the more your brain cells 'downregulate' by shutting down receptor sites. Continue along this slippery path for long enough and the effects of the stimulant become nothing like they used to be. No longer does that cup of coffee give you a rush of energy. Now all it does is relieve your ever-increasing fatigue. You need coffee just to feel normal, let alone good. You've been trying to cheat the system and it's fighting back. Crime, as far as falsely stimulating your neurotransmitters are concerned, doesn't pay.

Unfortunately, by the time you realise this and stop using the substance, your body's chemistry doesn't give you an unconditional pardon. Instead, it punishes you with withdrawal. In effect, the withdrawal period is the time it takes from the moment you quit using stimulants until your neurons 'upregulate' to hear your neurotransmitters' normal speaking voice once again. In the case of caffeine this is only a matter of days. For nicotine or heroin it can take weeks.

Essential Fats: Getting the Message

So far we've been talking about 'talking' – the way neurotransmitters deliver messages. Now let's look more closely at 'listening' – the neuron that receives the message. These neurons are surrounded by an insulating layer, called the myelin sheath, which is roughly 75 per cent fat, a quarter of it cholesterol. Embedded within this sheath are the receptor sites – we can think of them in this context as the ears receiving the messages. So, to get the message, and to prevent short-circuits in the brain (as happens in multiple sclerosis), you need a good supply of essential fats, also known as essential fatty acids (EFAs). You'll find out about these in detail in 'Natural High Basics', page 28.

Looking even closer at the myelin sheath (see below), we find that it is made out of a nutrient called a *phospholipid*, with two EFAs attached. It is

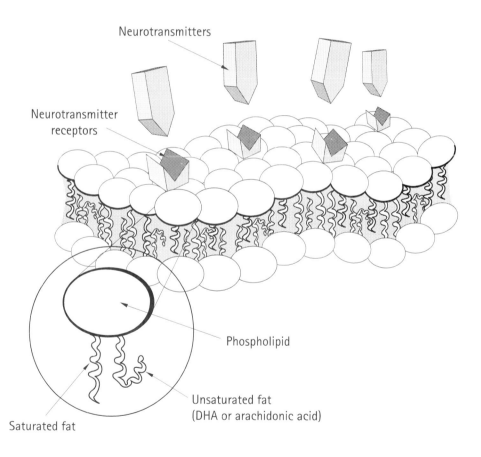

Neurotransmitters

Neurotransmitter receptors

Phospholipid

Unsaturated fat (DHA or arachidonic acid)

Saturated fat

The myelin sheath surrounding neurons is composed of phospholipids and fats

this combination of a phospholipid and two fatty acids that stops the cell from short-circuiting. These, too, will be discussed in the next chapter, on page 30, where we'll see how they, with EFAs, can actually keep us high.

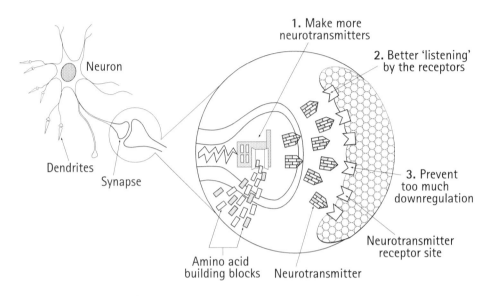

Diet and supplementation can improve neurotransmission in three ways

Three Ways to Get Your Brain Singing

Putting together everything you've learnt so far, you'll see that there are three possible ways of influencing or enhancing your neurotransmitter balance, and hence your mood and mind. We will describe each process so you can see how it works. All the suggestions for reaching a natural high are based on these simple principles.

1. Better talking

'Better talking' means making large enough quantities of the neurotransmitters you need. This means supplying the body and brain with the nutrients (in most cases, amino acids) that are the building blocks of the desired neurotransmitter.

For example, Jane doesn't eat a very well-balanced diet. She's lacking the amino acid tryptophan. As a consequence she is often depressed. She improves her diet and supplements tryptophan (or its cousin, 5-hydroxytryptophan – see page 108 for more details). As her serotonin levels improve, so too does her mood.

2. Better listening

'Better listening' means ensuring your brain's receptors are in tiptop condition. This means consuming optimal amounts of the building materials for these receptor sites – EFAs, especially omega-3s, and phospholipids, which are explained in more detail in the next chapter.

Jane starts to eat more fish, high in omega-3 fats, and adds a spoonful of lecithin granules, high in phospholipids, to her breakfast. Her mood becomes more stable and she starts to experience a consistently high level of mental energy.

3. Better talking *and* listening

If you consistently consume the right amounts of the right nutrients, and so maintain an optimal balance of neurotransmitters and 'receptive' receptors, you'll be preventing your body from needing to downregulate and therefore becoming tolerant. But using and abusing various substances means the body over-compensates by downregulation.

Jane used to go to parties and take Ecstasy (MDMA). She felt great because large amounts of serotonin were quickly released into her synapses. Unfortunately this was followed by serotonin depletion, leaving her tired and depressed the next day. Repeated use of Ecstasy soon caused her serotonin receptors to downregulate.

Jane learned that eating tryptophan-rich foods and taking the right supplements could replenish her serotonin stores. Now, she eats a great diet, takes the 'natural high' supplements mentioned above, meditates and exercises regularly. These keep her brain 'well-tuned' and because she feels good most of the time she has no desire for stimulants such as Ecstasy.

Having this perfect balance allows you to be naturally high most of the time, and rise to the inevitable stresses and challenges of life without getting unnecessarily anxious or depressed.

Congratulations – you've now completed your introduction to brain chemistry. You will see how every 'unnatural' substance we use gives us a short-term boost and a long-term burnout via tolerance, addiction and withdrawal, and how the secret to being naturally high is to tune up your neurotransmitters using specific natural, healthy and non-addictive nutrients and herbs.

NATURAL HIGH BASICS

W E'VE SEEN that if you want to be naturally high, the first step is to scout out the best food going. Optimum nutrition will help to keep your neurotransmitters in balance, and you in control of mind and mood.

It has been scientifically proven that following the principles of optimum nutrition can:

▶ Improve your mood
▶ Increase your energy
▶ Boost IQ scores
▶ Reduce stress
▶ Increase mental and physical stamina
▶ Enhance your concentration and memory

We'll be looking at all the nutrients in turn in this chapter, finishing off with a list of the basics that will get you – and keep you – high.

So where do you find the top-quality fuel and building materials that help you think and feel your best? For fuel, look to carbohydrates, while for building materials you'll need the fats and amino acids that make up protein.

The Power of Protein

Protein is vital. Since almost all neurotransmitters are made from it, you can influence how you feel by giving yourself the ideal quantity and quality of protein. By taking this in an easily absorbed form it can be put to good use by your body and brain. The better the quality and 'usability' of the protein you eat, the less you actually need in order to be optimally nourished.

The quality of a protein is determined by its balance of amino acids. Though there are twenty-three amino acids from which the body can build everything, from a neurotransmitter to a neuron, you actually need to eat only the eight so-called 'essential' amino acids, because the body can make the rest from these. The better the balance of amino acids – expressed as a unit called an NPU, which stands for net protein usability – the better use you can make of the protein.

The chart below shows the top individual foods and food combinations in terms of NPUs, or protein quality. Combining legumes with rice is a great way of increasing protein content. It also shows how much of a food, or food combination, you need to eat to get 20g of protein. A man needs to eat the equivalent of three to four of the indicated servings, while a woman needs to eat two to three.

A typical day's allotment of protein for a man might therefore include an egg for breakfast (10g), a 200g (7oz) salmon steak for lunch (40g) and a serving of beans with dinner (20g).

For a vegetarian, a typical day might be a small tub of yoghurt and a heaped tablespoon of seeds on an oat-based cereal (20g) for breakfast, and a 275g serving of tofu (20g), and vegetable steam-fry, served with either a cup of quinoa (20g), or a serving of beans with rice (20g) as part of dinner. The trick for vegetarians is to eat 'seed' foods – that is, foods that would grow if you planted them. These include seeds, nuts, beans, lentils, peas, corn or the germ of grains such as wheat or oat. 'Flower' foods, such as broccoli or cauliflower, are also relatively rich in protein.

Note that the cup measures indicated in the chart below and opposite are Imperial.

PACKED WITH PROTEIN: THE TOP 24

FOOD	PERCENTAGE OF CALORIES AS PROTEIN	HOW MUCH FOR 20G PROTEIN	PROTEIN QUALITY (NPU)
Grains/Pulses			
Quinoa	16	100g (3½ oz)/1 cup dry weight	Excellent
Tofu	40	275g (10 oz)/1 packet	Reasonable
Corn	4	500g (1 lb 2 oz)/3 cups cooked weight	Reasonable

Food	Percentage of calories as protein	How much for 20g Protein	Protein quality (NPU)
Brown rice	5	400g (14 oz)/3 cups cooked weight	Excellent
Chickpeas	22	115g (4 oz)/0.66 cup cooked weight	Reasonable
Lentils	28	85g (3 oz)/1 cup cooked weight	Reasonable
Fish/meat			
Tuna, canned	61	85g (3 oz)/1 small tin	Excellent
Cod	60	35g (1¼ oz)/1 very small piece	Excellent
Salmon	50	100g (3½ oz)/1 very small piece	Excellent
Sardines	49	100g (3½ oz)/1 grilled	Excellent
Chicken	63	75g (2½ oz)/1 small roasted breast	Excellent
Nuts/seeds			
Sunflower seeds	15	185g (6½ oz)/1 cup	Reasonable
Pumpkin seeds	21	75g (2½ oz)/0.5 cup	Reasonable
Cashew nuts	12	115g (4 oz)/1 cup	Reasonable
Almonds	13	115g (4 oz)/1 cup	Reasonable
Eggs/dairy			
Eggs	34	115g (4 oz)/2 medium	Excellent
Yoghurt, natural	22	450g (1 lb)/3 small pots	Excellent
Cottage cheese	49	125g (4½ oz)/1 small pot	Excellent
Vegetables			
Peas, frozen	26	250g (9 oz)/2 cups	Reasonable
Other beans	20	200g (7 oz)/2 cups	Reasonable
Broccoli	50	40g (1½ oz)/0.5 cup	Reasonable
Spinach	49	40g (1½ oz)/0.66 cup	Reasonable
Combinations			
Lentils and rice	18	125g (4½ oz)/small cup dry weight	Excellent
Beans and rice	15	125g (4½ oz)/small cup dry weight	Excellent

Running on Carbohydrates

The best fuel for all body cells, including brain cells, is glucose. Most carbohydrates – bread, cereals, fruits and vegetables – break down into this simple sugar during digestion. In a sedentary day, up to 50 per cent of the glucose you consume goes to power the brain. Even though it weighs only 1.3kg (3 lb), the brain is the most sugar-hungry organ of the body.

Again, you need both the right quantity and quality of carbohydrate. For the brain to have a steady supply of glucose, it has to be slowly released from food into the bloodstream. The top brain fuel foods are therefore 'slow-release' carbohydrates – those that gradually release their energy-giving glucose into the bloodstream. And there's an easy way to determine which carbohydrates fall into this category: the glycaemic index (GI). This ranks foods by how much your blood sugar increases in the 2 to 3 hours after eating them. Foods with a low GI include complex carbohydrates, such as whole, unrefined grains, some fruits, and almost all vegetables. For an ideal diet, choose the low GI foods that score under 50 in the chart on pages 27 and 28.

A typical day's allowance of low-GI carbohydrates might include a wholegrain cereal such as oat flakes with an apple, pear or berries in the morning, a wholegrain sandwich with salad or vegetables for lunch, and some wholewheat or buckwheat pasta, rice or beans with dinner.

Another way to slow the release of carbohydrate in food is to combine it with protein. So you could have a salmon steak with brown basmati rice, chicken with boiled new potatoes or tofu with wholewheat pasta.

Fats for the Brain

Essential fats are important for mind and mood. In fact, 60 per cent of the brain is made from fat, and essential fats make a big difference to brain cell communication. So, if you want to be naturally high you need to ensure an optimal intake of them. We estimate that around 30 per cent of the calories in your diet should come from fat.

The complete glycaemic index (GI) of foods
For an ideal diet, choose the low GI foods that score under 50.

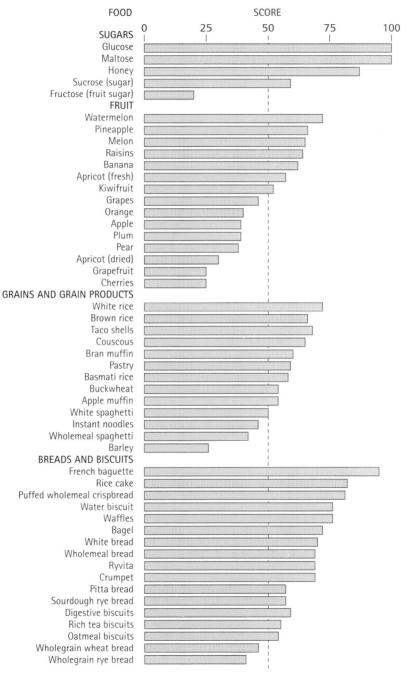

The complete glycaemic index (GI) of foods.
For an ideal diet, choose the low GI foods that score under 50.

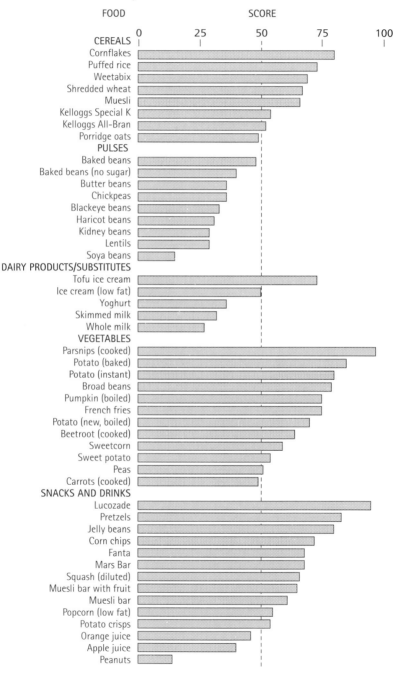

FOOD

SCORE

| | 0 | 25 | 50 | 75 | 100 |

The average diet consists of 40 per cent fat, mainly from meat, dairy products and junk foods, which are high in saturated and hydrogenated fats. These hydrogenated fats may sound good on food labels, where they're often described as *polyunsaturated hydrogenated* vegetable oils. But in truth, hydrogenating a fat makes it like a saturated fat, no longer able to do all the wonderful things that the unprocessed (essential) polyunsaturated fats can do. Even worse, while they can be incorporated into the brain, they don't work. The net result is that people who fill themselves up with high-fat junk foods literally numb their thinking processes. In other words, the wrong kind of fats literally lowers your intelligence and worsens your mood.

Alpha and Omega: the essential fats

The reverse is also true. If you increase your intake of the right kinds of polyunsaturated fats, your mind and mood will get a tremendous boost. These are omega-3 and omega-6 essential fatty acids or EFAs, and you need equal amounts of these in your diet (see the figure below). Omega-3 fats are found in flaxseeds (also called linseeds) and in fish, especially oily coldwater fish such as herring, mackerel, tuna and salmon. Omega-6 fats are found in sesame, sunflower and pumpkin seeds and oils.

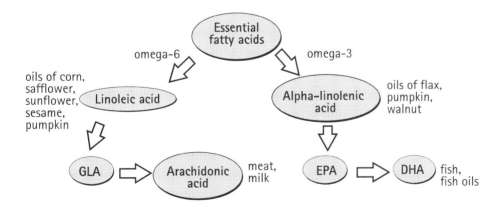

The brain's essential fats and their sources

Since seeds are also a wonderful source of protein, minerals and vitamin E, we recommend that you eat a heaped tablespoon of seeds every day. In practical terms, an ideal mix would be half flaxseeds, with the remaining half made up of sesame, sunflower, hemp and pumpkin seeds. Since some of these seeds are quite tough, you will get more nutrients out of them by grinding them in a coffee grinder and then sprinkling them on your morning cereal, or in soups, salads or casseroles.

Essential fats are easily damaged and lose their nutritional value if heated or stored too long, especially if they are exposed to light. So the best way to protect the oils in seeds is to keep them in a tightly sealed glass jar in the fridge.

In addition to your daily heaped tablespoon of the ground seed mix, adding one of the following will help you achieve an optimal intake of omega-3 fats:

▶ A serving of an oily fish three times a week

or

▶ A daily fish oil supplement providing 400mg of EPA plus DHA

or (for strict vegetarians)

▶ A daily dessertspoon of flaxseed oil

or

▶ An additional heaped tablespoon of ground or soaked flaxseeds.

You can also buy organic cold-pressed seed oil blends that provide both omega-3 and omega-6 fats. These are great to use in salad dressings, in preference to olive oil (which only provides 8 per cent omega-6) and instead of butter, drizzled on vegetables or other food after cooking. Never use these polyunsaturated oils for frying though.

Essential fats need to be in balance in your brain. EFAs that hang off phospholipid molecules in the brain (see page 19) are either DHA (a type of omega-3 fat) or arachidonic acid (an omega-6 fat). Arachidonic acid is found in animal meat, squid, eggs and milk and can also be made from those omega-6 fats found in seeds, although you only tend to make what you need from these seeds. Too much arachidonic acid isn't good for you, which is why a diet high in meat and low in fish can worsen mental and emotional performance. So a good balance is really key.

Phospholipids: the insulation experts

In the last chapter we also met another kind of 'intelligent' fat in your brain – the recently discovered phospholipids. Phospholipids are there in abundance because they make up the insulating layer, or myelin, of all nerves. There are two kinds – phosphatidyl choline and phosphatidyl serine. These are classified as smart nutrients because, without a doubt, they enhance your mood, mind and mental performance. Phospholipids also protect against age-related memory decline and Alzheimer's disease.

Although the body can make them, getting extra phospholipids from food is doubly beneficial. Egg yolk is the richest source of phospholipids in the average diet. But since egg phobia set in, amid fears that dietary cholesterol was a major cause of heart disease, the average intake of phospholipids has dropped dramatically. Significantly, cases of Alzheimer's have rocketed. (The American Heart Association now states that you can eat up to seven eggs a week.)

Lecithin is an excellent source of phospholipids, and widely available in health-food stores as either granules or capsules. 'Lecithin is practically a wonder-drug as far as cognitive impairment is concerned,' says Dr Dharma Singh Khalsa, author of *Brain Longevity*, and an expert in nutrition and its role in preventing memory decline. You'll need about 5g of lecithin a day, or half this if you take 'high-PC' (phosphatidyl choline) lecithin, as a natural high basic. The easiest and cheapest way to take this is to add a tablespoon of lecithin, or a heaped teaspoon of high-PC lecithin, to your cereal in the morning. Or you can take lecithin supplements. Most capsules provide 1200mg, so you would need four a day. By the way, lecithin doesn't make you fat. In fact, quite the opposite: it helps the body digest fat.

Water, water . . .

Two-thirds of your body, and almost half of your brain, is made of water. Obviously, this makes it vital for optimal brain and body function. Ageing, for instance, is a dehydrating process: as you age the water content in your body and brain decreases. So drinking enough water can slow down the ageing process. But how much do you need? The ideal daily intake is around 2 litres (3½ pints), and more if you live in a hot climate or exercise a lot.

Fruits and vegetables are around 90 per cent water, and provide it in a form that is very easy for the body to use. (They are also, of course, a great source of vitamins and minerals.) These foods can provide a litre (1¾ pints) of water if you eat enough of them, leaving just an extra litre a day to be obtained from water or diluted juices, and herb or fruit teas. Alcohol, tea and coffee are diuretics and flush water from the body, as well as robbing it of valuable minerals. So we don't recommend them as sources of fluid intake.

It's easy to up your water intake. One way is to keep a jug or bottle of filtered or spring water on your desk at work. Fill it up in the morning and drink it all by the time you go home. Keep a bottle of spring water in your bedroom too, so you can drink some first thing in the morning.

Mopping up with Antioxidants

Oxygen is the ultimate 'essential' – a few minutes without it and you're dead. We need to breathe it, of course, and 'burning' food with oxygen gives our bodies energy.

The trouble is, whenever we make energy, we also make toxic by-products called oxidants – a whole bucketful of them a year. And many of us produce far more than this. One puff of a cigarette, for example, lets loose a trillion oxidant molecules in the smoker. Exhaust fumes, pollution, fried and browned food and exposure to the sun can be equally disastrous.

Oxidants are the major cause of the ageing process. They attack brain cells and are largely responsible for the decline in their number as we age. Essential fats and neurotransmitters are also highly susceptible to damage by oxidants.

How can you keep them at bay? Increase your intake of antioxidants, a family of nutrients with the power to mop up oxidants, and so reverse the ageing process. Top antioxidants include prunes, raisins, blueberries and blackberries, while kale, spinach, strawberries, raspberries, plums, broccoli and alfalfa sprouts aren't far behind.

These, and other fresh fruits and vegetables, are the kind of foods you need to eat every day to stay young and energetic. Make sure your daily supplement programme contains significant quantities of antioxidants, especially if you are older, live in a polluted city or have any other unavoidable exposure to oxidants. A comprehensive antioxidant supplement, paired with a good multivitamin and mineral tablet, is the best way to do this. Most reputable supplement companies produce formulas containing a combination of the following nutrients – vitamin A, beta-carotene, vitamin E, vitamin C, zinc, selenium, glutathione and cysteine, plus plant-based antioxidants such as anthocyanidins from a source such as bilberry or pycnogenol.

Live and Kicking: Vitamins and Minerals

When it comes to how you think and feel, vitamins and minerals are magicians. They can work real wonders in the brain, where they're used the most. B vitamins, for instance, can stave off depression, anxiety, stress, confusion, fatigue, mental dullness and emotional fragility, and can even boost IQ. The minerals magnesium (Mg), iron (Fe), zinc (Zn), manganese (Mn) and chromium (Cr), plus antioxidant nutrients, especially vitamin C, are also vital for brain power and health. If you want to make sure your body can produce just what it needs at any given moment, you need to eat foods rich in vital vitamins and minerals, as well as supplementing your diet.

Unconvinced of their power? Consider this research. Ninety school-children were assigned to one of three groups: one received a multivitamin and mineral supplement, one received an identical-looking placebo, one received nothing. After 7 months the IQ of those taking the supplements had increased by a staggering 9 points![1] A 5-point increase would get half the learning-disabled children out of special schools and back to normal schooling.

These vital vitamins and minerals are found mostly in whole and 'live' food, so it's these you should concentrate on. Whole foods – foods you could pluck out of a tree or pull out of the ground, or eat as they are in nature – include beans, lentils, seeds, nuts, whole grains such as brown rice, wholewheat bread or pasta, as well as fresh fruits, vegetables, fish, meat and eggs. Seeds are especially rich in minerals such as calcium, magnesium, zinc and iron as well as fibre.

As it hasn't been injected with preservatives, whole food goes off quicker. The trick is to eat it before it does! Fresh fruits and vegetables are much richer in nutrients and antioxidants than dried foods that are stored for months before you eat them. So search for fruits and vegetables that are *really* fresh – farmers' markets and organic suppliers can be good sources.

The fresh stuff isn't the whole story, though. To achieve optimum health and nutrition, you need to 'eat right *and* take a multivitamin', as a recent headline in the *New England Journal of Medicine* editorial had it.[2] 'The evidence suggests,' stated the journal, 'that people who take such supplements and their children are healthier.' A good, high-strength multivitamin plus 1 to 3g of vitamin C a day is your insurance policy for a natural high.

Natural High Basics

▶ Eat three servings a day of top-quality protein foods – fish, lean white meat (free range), egg, soya, quinoa or combinations of beans, lentils and grains.
▶ Choose low-GI carbohydrates such as whole grains, vegetables and most fruits, and stay away from sugar and refined foods.
▶ Combine protein with carbohydrate.
▶ Avoid hydrogenated fats and reduce your intake of saturated fats from meat, dairy produce and junk food.
▶ Eat fish three times a week instead of meat, or take fish oil supplements.

▶ Have a heaped tablespoon of ground seeds every day.

▶ Use cold-pressed seed oils in salad dressings.

▶ Drink at least a litre (1¾ pints) of water, if not two, a day, as water or in diluted juices and herb or fruit teas.

▶ Minimise your intake of tea, coffee and alcohol.

▶ Eat lots of antioxidant-rich fruits and vegetables – at least five servings a day.

▶ Make sure most of your diet is made up of whole foods and fresh foods.

▶ Have a tablespoon of lecithin every day.

▶ Take these supplements daily:

  – A high-strength multivitamin and mineral

  – 1 to 3g of vitamin C

  – An antioxidant formula.

PART TWO

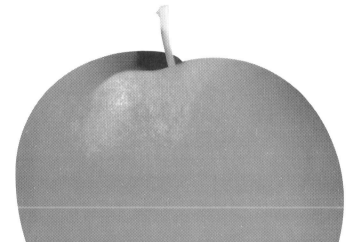

NATURAL
ALTERNATIVES

◀4▶

RELAXANTS

CHILLING OUT at the end of the day or at the weekend feels great. After all you've worked hard, you're tired, you need a break – and what better way to relax than in a hot bath, or with a favourite CD, a good book or the company of friends? These alone can be great highs.

For a lot of us, though, relaxing is more than just a pleasure: it's vital for our health, and we may even need to relearn how to do it. We're *stressed*.

Stress is pervasive and potentially harmful. For some of us it even seems to be a way of life. Understanding it and finding ways of dealing with it effectively are key to living on a natural high. We'll be looking at how stress affects our minds and bodies, as well as at some of the common substances we use to deal with it – even though they are ineffective. We'll examine the natural anti-stressors that *do* work, some of them able to take us into states of blissful relaxation. You'll even see how stress can be turned to your own advantage.

The Anatomy of Stress

Can you relate to this scenario? It's Monday morning, and you barely have enough time to drop your daughter at school on your way to work. Just as you're both ready to leave the house, she complains of a tummy ache. You have an important meeting at 9 am, and soon everyone will be waiting for you. She does look a bit ill, though, so you stop and take her temperature, delaying you further. Your mind races: 'Should I stay home with her? Is there someone I can leave her with today?' You have suddenly become a victim of forces beyond your control, creating a one-way ticket to stress that wreaks havoc on mind and body.

Welcome to life in the twenty-first century. We feel pressured to keep up with jobs, family and the myriad responsibilities of everyday life. Hardly a moment goes by when we are not subject to some form of stress. Many of us end up anxious, depressed and exhausted – the price we pay for our complex lifestyles. Are we doomed to move faster and faster, like mice in a maze seeking the elusive cheese, or is there a realistic solution to the ever-growing problem of stress?

Stress Check

We need a certain amount of stress to keep us motivated. But when it takes over our lives, it can adversely affect us. How do you score on the stress scale? This quiz will help you recognise some of the signs and see where you fit in the stress continuum.

Score 1 for each 'yes' answer.

How Stressed Are You?	Yes	No
Do you have difficulty relaxing ?	☐	☐
Do you find yourself feeling irritable?	☐	☐
Do you worry about little events of the day and are you unable to shut your mind off?	☐	☐
Do you smoke or drink excessively (especially by others' standards)?	☐	☐
Are you competitive and aggressive in the things you do?	☐	☐
Do you find it hard to relate to people?	☐	☐
Do you find you are impatient with others?	☐	☐
Do you eat quickly?	☐	☐
Do you take on too much?	☐	☐
Do you have difficulty delegating?	☐	☐
Do you have aching limbs or recurrent headaches?	☐	☐
Do you have a dry mouth and sweaty palms?	☐	☐
Do you feel a lack of interest in sex?	☐	☐
Are your muscles tense?	☐	☐
Do you have problems sleeping?	☐	☐

If your score is:

Below 5: You're in fine shape, able to take life in your stride. But perhaps you'd like to be super-calm and super-relaxed. Check out this chapter for some fun ideas.

5 to 10: You are quite stressed; pay attention to these warning signs. This is the only body you have: treat it well. You'll see how to do this in the following pages.

More than 10: You are very stressed: clean up your act before it has serious consequences. Read on to find out how.

Why do we have such a strong reaction to stress? It's how we evolved to cope with emergencies: stress mobilises the body's 'fight or flight' response. The brain signals the tiny almond-shaped adrenal glands perched on top of the kidneys, to produce the stress hormones adrenalin and cortisol. This increases our breathing and heart rates, elevates our blood pressure and raises our blood sugar levels, preparing our body for either self-defence or escape.

Our particular stressors may be modern, but the stress response is quite ancient – and worked fine when we were running from fierce predators at the dawn of human existence. However, as much as we'd like to, we can't run from our boss, our stalled car or the ringing telephone. So, unlike our ancestors, we have no way of burning off this excess energy.

On top of this physical burden, we store mental images of the traumatic event for years afterwards. Popping up in our memory in response to similar events, or even at random moments, our minds and bodies react as if the incident were occurring right now. This re-creates the stress response, producing anxiety all over again. In contrast, animals in the wild will actually go through a series of movements that disperse the energy and complete the stress cycle right away. Psychologist Peter Levine does a wonderful job of exploring these ideas in his book, *Waking the Tiger Within*.

This brings us to the fact that much of our problem exists in the mind!

It's all in your head

'. . . There is nothing either good or bad but thinking makes it so' (*Hamlet*, Act 2, Scene 2). Shakespeare had a point. The truth is, unless your house burns down or someone dies, most stresses are not disasters. Thinking they are, however, can easily overwhelm you. As we said, the problem doesn't even have to be real or present – it can be in the past or the future, or *only* in the mind.

When we worry about an upcoming job interview or a blind date, we may find ourselves with a dry mouth, sweaty palms or queasy stomach. We might become fidgety, restless and pace about, or have difficulty falling asleep. Our nerves or anxiety are our *emotional response* to stress. Incidentally, anxiety is not always a bad thing. That feeling of apprehension, the gnawing feeling in the pit of our stomach that 'something is wrong', is a natural warning signal. We have all used it as a motivator at times, to study for final exams, or to pay our bills on time. When it works overtime, though, it causes problems.

In addition to the usual addictive substances, for probably the first time in history people in the West are also addicted to stress. This is not to say we love it, but, just as one cup of coffee begs another, and a cigarette leads to the next, stress begets more stress. Many of us end up not only addicted to the substances that we take, but literally addicted to our own stress neurotransmitters and hormones! We get the same physiological high from the dopamine and endorphin-enhancing effects of adrenalin that we do from a stimulant. Adrenalin keeps us going, but after a while it's the only thing that does. We're running on empty. Then, when we finally take some time off, we collapse in a heap – depleted, depressed and exhausted. We may feel blue or bored. Our 'get up and go' has 'got up and gone'. We need, in short, to relax.

Fight or Flight – The Stress Response

Nobel prize winner Dr Hans Selye, the father of stress research, proposed three stages to this stress response. This 'General Adaptation Syndrome' (GAS) consists of alarm, adaptation, and finally exhaustion (see opposite). His model is useful in helping you see where you are in the stress cycle, and what to do about it.

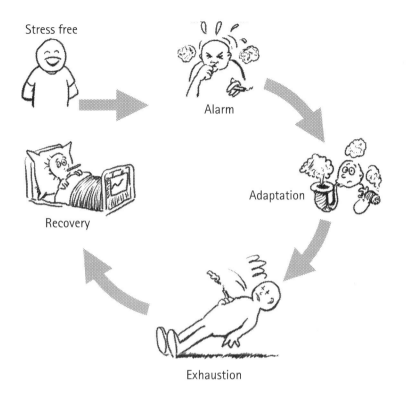

The general adaptation syndrome, from a stress-free state to exhaustion and recovery

The alarm stage

When you are first stressed (the alarm phase) the brain signals the adrenal glands to produce about 40 hormones, most importantly adrenalin and cortisol. The adrenalin effect kicks in immediately, while the cortisol one lasts for longer. These both give a boost to your blood sugar. In fact, the average 'adrenal rush' of a commuter stuck in traffic supplies enough glucose to keep him running for a mile. The adrenals also release the hormone DHEA (dehydroepiandrosterone), which helps maintain energy and resistance to stress.

As a result of this rapid deployment of adrenalin, cortisol and DHEA, we have more oxygen and sugar available, push more blood to the brain and muscles, and are instantly more alert. In fact, many people will create stress in their lives just to experience this stimulation.

Adaptation stage

When the body needs to continue its defence mechanism beyond the initial 'fight or flight' response, it enters the adaptation phase. Cortisol and DHEA have a reciprocal relationship, so as cortisol levels go up, DHEA levels fall. We start to feel the effects of long-term stress, with increasing anxiety, fatigue and mood swings.

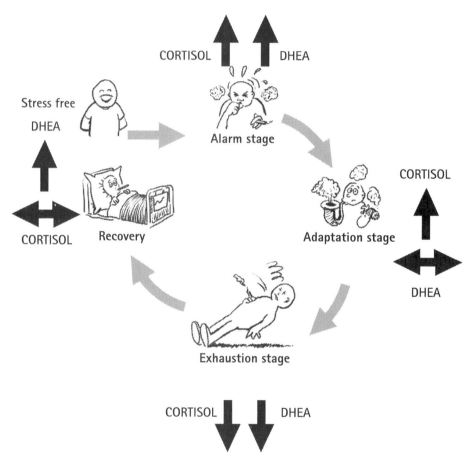

The stress cycle, and how hormone levels fluctuate

Exhaustion stage

When we become stuck in the stress response or when it becomes chronic, we enter the dangerous territory of the exhaustion phase. No longer can we produce the necessary cortisol to respond to stress. Our DHEA levels plummet. We become depleted of vitamins, including vitamin C, the B vitamins, and essential minerals such as magnesium. Our energy plummets and, since adrenalin is derived from the 'feel-good' neurotransmitter dopamine (see page 14), excess adrenalin demands lead to dopamine deficiency. Consequently our emotions can take a dive into depression.

The good news is that you can recover – and we're going to tell you how (on page 55).

The Costs of Stress

The extra energy liberated by adrenal stimulation comes at a high cost. In the short term, stress does the following:

▶ Suppresses the immune system, increasing the risk of infections
▶ Slows down the body's rate of repair
▶ Slows down the metabolism
▶ Robs the body of vital nutrients.

There can be physical symptoms:

▶ Recurrent headaches
▶ Vague aches and pains
▶ Dizziness
▶ Heartburn
▶ Muscle tension
▶ Dry mouth

▶ Excessive perspiration
▶ Pounding heart
▶ Insomnia
▶ Fatigue.

In the long term, stress:

▶ Promotes rapid ageing
▶ Leads to weight gain
▶ Increases the risk of developing osteoporosis, high blood pressure, heart disease, cancer and digestive problems.

On an emotional level, when our brain runs out of feel-good chemicals, we experience the following:

▶ Anxiety, fear, restlessness
▶ Irritability, anger
▶ Depression
▶ Insecurity
▶ Loss of libido
▶ Impaired memory and concentration
▶ Excessive smoking and/or drinking.

Blood sugar blues

Adrenalin and cortisol activity isn't the only danger when we're heavily stressed. Our blood sugar, or glucose, levels rise too, then abruptly fall. This is because both adrenalin and cortisol temporarily release stores of sugar into the bloodstream. You can get the same effect from a stimulant such as coffee, or by eating sugar. Then there's the rebound and your blood sugar level plummets. This is serious, because 20 per cent of the body's entire intake of glucose fuels the brain, the first area to suffer when

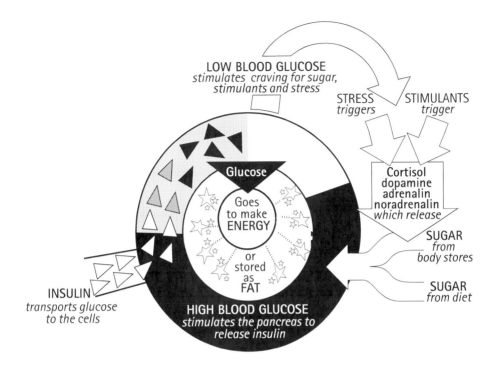

The vicious cycle of sugar, stress and stimulants

glucose is scarce. A dip in blood sugar may leave you feeling tired, nervous, foggy, or irritable, impatient and temperamental. And to relieve this discomfort you may reach for a doughnut, cola or a cigarette. So you end up feeding a vicious cycle.

The good news is that a proper diet and specific nutrients can break the cycle. For details see Chapter 3, on carbohydrate needs.

Chemical Coping: Drink, Dope and Downers

So much for the body's pharmacopoeia of beneficial and not-so-beneficial solutions to stress – what about the chemicals in the cupboard that we take to cope? When we're stressed, irritable or worried, most of us relax with a drink, a joint or even a prescribed tranquilliser such as Valium (diazepam) or Xanax (alprazolam). All of these take the edge off.

You know how it goes? You've just finished a hard day at the office, with some take-home work to prepare for tomorrow's meeting. You get on the road and sit in barely moving traffic for the next 40 minutes, come home to an equally harried spouse and kids vying for your attention. All you want to do is have a drink and forget about everything. . . . Or you're a student, with a paper due, and your computer just wiped out an entire afternoon's work. A joint looks really good to you right now. . . . Or you just found out you owe back taxes, and, while you don't know whose fault it is, you're the one who has to come up with the funds. Where is that bottle of Valium?

These scenarios may be realistic – but can we say the same about the solutions? The substances people so often take to chill out have their share of downsides. Let's see how they work and what those downsides are. They include:

▶ Alcohol
▶ Tranquillisers
▶ Cannabis
▶ Nicotine.

As you will see, each of these exert their relaxing effects by boosting these brain chemicals:

▶ GABA, the relaxing neurotransmitter
▶ Dopamine, the 'feel-good' neurotransmitter
▶ Endorphins, our natural euphoriant.

All liquored up: alcohol examined

For at least 6,000 years of recorded history, human beings have been enjoying alcohol. Today, it plays a pivotal role in society and in economics, with 120 million alcoholic drinks consumed each week in the UK alone.

What happens when you take a drink? Within minutes, that first glass of the evening is loosening you up, lowering your inhibitions, and putting you in a cheery and gregarious mood. This is due to the release of dopamine, which stimulates you, followed by endorphins, which make you feel high, and then GABA, which makes you relax. The alcohol also gives your blood sugar a boost. Sounds good, doesn't it? It feels good too, and that's why we do it. This pleasant effect usually lasts for an hour or so.

Several drinks later, though, you might notice you're feeling irritable, depressed or even hostile (or others will). Your thinking and memory may get fuzzy. You could end up unsure of where you are, whom you're with and why you're there. You might then get sleepy or, on a bad night, pass out.

A 'hangover' – nausea, headache, spaciness or stomach upset – may greet you the following morning. You may also have forgotten much of what happened the night before, a phenomenon known as a 'blackout'. This can be a serious problem if you've really abandoned your inhibitions. You may wonder whether the good time was worth it.

Here are some sobering statistics on drinking:

▶ A recent British study noted that alcohol use cost £2 billion (US$3.3 billion) in lost wages each year, most of which resulted from work missed because of hangovers. Hangover-induced absenteeism and poor job performance costs the US economy about $148 billion (£90 billion) a year.

▶ Researchers found that people with hangovers posed a danger to themselves and others long after their blood alcohol levels had returned to normal, suggesting that hangovers could be more insidious than actual inebriation.

Why Alcohol is Bad News

Short term

▶ Impaired memory: You're not sure where you left your keys, or your car, or who you flirted with (or more) the night before.

▶ Blackouts: You can recall nothing due to the toxic by-products of alcohol – the information was not stored.

▶ Impaired sexual function.

▶ Inappropriate behaviour, dehydration, and accidents – including fatal ones.

▶ Morning-after hangover.

Long term

▶ Addiction. Though the stimulation effect may feel good, the brain seeks internal balance or *homeostasis*. When you keep pushing the brain to release a neurotransmitter, it responds by 'downregulating' – that is, over time, you will need to drink more to keep getting the same effect.

▶ Long-term alcohol use can lead to a host of health problems: gastritis, ulcers, liver problems including cirrhosis (where scar tissue replaces liver cells), pancreatic disease, and permanent brain and nerve damage.

▶ Pregnant women who abuse alcohol can seriously damage their unborn infants.

▶ Depletion of neurotransmitters and nutrients.

▶ Chronic alcoholic patients can suffer convulsions from a life-threatening condition called 'the DTs' (delirium tremens), caused by alcohol withdrawal.

Sedatives and tranquillisers: 'mother's little helpers'

From the early 1900s until the mid-1950s, barbiturates such as phenobarbital and Seconal were the mainstay for treating anxiety and insomnia. Unfortunately, they were also associated with thousands of suicides, accidental deaths, both of children who took them and adults who overdosed on them, widespread dependency and abuse, and chemical incompatibility with other drugs and alcohol. By 1954, they were being replaced by the new, 'non-addictive' meprobamate (Miltown) as the calming agent of choice. They turned out to be as addictive as the old drugs. Then, the 1960s introduced the currently popular benzodiazepines: diazepam (Valium), chlordiazepoxide (Librium), clonazapine (Klonopin) and the shorter-acting alprazolam (Xanax) or temazepam (Restoril). In the UK 16 million prescriptions are written annually for these so-called 'minor tranquillisers' to treat anxiety and insomnia. Their calming effect is due to their action on the receptors for the inhibitory neurotransmitter GABA (gamma aminobutyric acid). By increasing GABA activity, the benzodiazepines tend to dull both awareness and overall brain activity. So they calm your anxiety but dull your senses.

Mary is a case in point.

When she was in her thirties, Mary found herself stuck in an unhappy marriage, and with a young child. Seeing no escape, she was taking large doses of Valium to shut out the pain. One day, while filling yet another prescription for Mary, the pharmacist said, 'In case you don't know it, you're addicted. Speak to me when you're ready to stop.' This was Mary's wake-up call.

In shocked response, Mary simply stopped the drug cold. She was too ashamed to face the pharmacist, who would have advised a slow withdrawal programme under medical supervision. Then, not knowing she was suffering from withdrawal symptoms, she simply, in her words, 'went crazy' for the next 2 months or so. It took that long for her brain to readjust itself.

What had happened was that the Valium had caused Mary's brain to down-regulate. It had adjusted to Valium's relaxing action. This led to extreme agitation (withdrawal) when she stopped it, until, in time, her brain readjusted itself. 'When I finally got my mind back, I decided to leave my husband. I never looked back. Nor did I ever dare take another tranquilliser,' declares Mary, now, at 48, a successful writer and a proud grandmother.

Fortunately for Mary, her pharmacist said the right thing. Many other prescription-drug addicts, however, will go for years having their prescription refilled in large, impersonal pharmacies, or will rotate between several different stores. Harried physicians who have little time to really listen to patients find it easier to renew a prescription than to deal with someone's symptoms. And the prospect of detoxification is a tough one for either of them to deal with.

Be very aware that if you are addicted to tranquillisers, withdrawal needs to be taken seriously.[1] It can be fatal if not done correctly and under medical supervision. See the Appendix, page 283, for details about how to come off them, and minimise withdrawal symptoms using safe, non-addictive herbal remedies.

Downsides of Benzodiazepines

▶ Tolerance: after taking them for some time, more is required to get the same effect.

▶ Forgetfulness, drowsiness, accident-proneness, social withdrawal.

▶ 'Rebound' anxiety as a result of withdrawal and insomnia.

▶ Hangover: grogginess the next morning, accidents caused not only right after ingestion, but the following day; undetected hangover effect.

▶ Addiction: must continue to take it just to stay 'even', and causes serious withdrawal effects upon quitting, including anxiety, insomnia, irritability, tremors, mental impairment, headaches – possibly even seizures and death.

Cannabis: from the Stone Age to the 'stoned' age

People in Asian and Middle Eastern countries have used marijuana (*Cannabis sativa*) as an intoxicant for thousands of years. With the birth of Islam, cannabis was embraced as the preferred psychoactive substance, replacing the Judaeo-Christian favourite, alcohol. Cannabis was later used in Western medicine for at least two millennia, until the early 1900s, when the use of pharmaceuticals largely replaced herbal medicines. It was finally declared illegal for medical use in the 1930s. During the 1960s and 1970s its use was rife in universities, communes and wherever young people gathered, and it became associated with youth culture. Today it is the most widely used of all illegal drugs.

How does it work? The immediate effects of smoking cannabis are mild euphoria and, often, drowsiness. Research shows that there are receptors for cannabis in the brain which lead to the release of the feel-good neurotransmitter dopamine. Cannabis' effects on judgement, coordination and short-term memory make it inadvisable to drive, operate heavy machinery or try to learn anything new while under its influence. This is due to the high concentration of cannabis receptors in both the hippocampus, the part of the brain that controls memory, and the cerebellum, which governs motor coordination. Moreover, these effects may actually last longer than those of alcohol. Research on the effects of driving under the influence of cannabis concludes that impairment persists for 4 to 8 hours, long after the subjective effects have worn off. Some 94 per cent of subjects fail roadside sobriety tests 90 minutes after smoking, while 60 per cent fail after 150 minutes.[2] Just as with alcohol and tranquillisers, the effects last longer than is easily recognised, resulting in needless accidents.

Up in smoke: side-effects

Researchers have shown that daily users, after several days of abstinence, continue to show subtle but measurable impairment in their mental processing. But it's not clear whether this after-the-fact impairment results from changes in the brain or is just a slow, continuous release of marijuana constituents that have been stored in the brain and fatty tissues.

Here's the experience of Gene, a 45-year-old, married, physical therapist.

I'd only smoked a hit or two every other day, but I had done it for years. I finally stopped smoking marijuana completely 8 months ago, and I feel a lot better. My work-outs have improved and my overall energy level is up. When I smoked, on the other hand, I would feel relaxed at first, but after an hour or so, my mood would dip. I'd get cranky, and want another hit. The next one wouldn't do it, though, so I gave up trying. The moodiness was probably due to a low blood sugar reaction – you know, 'the munchies'. Then I'd eat, so I put on weight, which I didn't need.

I finally decided I'd had enough of it all, and just quit. I became really irritable. Not only was I craving a smoke, but had to handle all kinds of emotional issues that were coming up, things I hadn't ever dealt with. Fortunately, I had some aromatherapy and herbal products that really helped cut the cravings and lift my mood. Eventually, after about 6 or 8 weeks, my moods evened out. Now, if I find myself wanting a joint to relax, I take a whiff of my aromatherapy oil or a dose of kava. Overall, I'm glad to be over the whole thing. Life feels more real to me now. My wife likes me better now, too. She says I'm more emotionally stable and available, and nicer to be with.

In our own observations, young people who smoked their way through high school (or even earlier) and continued to do so through young adulthood are more likely to have problems. They seem less able to cope with the challenges of everyday life, or be able to plan appropriately for their future. Their emotional development appears blunted: the marijuana fog may have prevented them from fully experiencing a complete range of emotions and relationships. Stoned on the hero's journey, they miss the passages necessary for growing up and accepting their place in the adult world.

Cannabis can also cause the same throat and lung irritation as tobacco, which is a known carcinogen. The existence of any other long-term problems resulting from its use remains a question, since there is no definitive research available.

Pitfalls of Pot

▶ Impairs coordination, judgement and short-term memory, which persists for 4 to 8 hours. May result in accidents.

▶ Mood swings, irritability due to low blood sugar reaction.

> ▶ Blunted emotional development in young people who are chronic users leading to problems in coping with everyday challenges, and planning their future.
>
> ▶ Throat and lung irritation, as with tobacco.

Relaxing Naturally – with Herbs

We have seen how drink, dope and downers work by promoting the relaxing neurotransmitter GABA, the feel-good neurotransmitter dopamine, and the endorphins, or euphoriants. However, they also lead to neurotransmitter and blood sugar imbalances that can get you into all kinds of trouble, from emotional and mental impairment to addiction. There are healthier natural choices that achieve the same goal, but without the negative effects.

While the ideal is to be stress-free and not in need of relaxants at all, the reality is that we do get stressed and need to restore balance. This means:

▶ Balancing your blood sugar
▶ Promoting release of GABA
▶ Supporting the release of dopamine and endorphins
▶ Supplying the appropriate nutrients to produce them.

Stress depletes the body of vital nutrients. The more stressed we are, the more quickly we become deficient, and the more of these nutrients we need. For example, we need B vitamins for a smoothly running nervous system and for adrenal hormone production. There are also certain minerals that have a relaxing effect on the body and emotions. Make sure that you are taking enough of the following: vitamins B1, B3, B6, B12, folic acid, calcium, magnesium and omega-3 fatty acids, such as fish or flax seed oil, especially under stressful conditions. Following the 'Natural High Basics' (see Chapter 3) will give you a solid basis on which to experience the full benefit of natural relaxants.

As we have seen, alcohol, cannabis and tranquillisers affect one or more of these keys to relaxation. As we saw in the cases of Mary and Gene, they create significant rebound effects as relaxation is followed by irritability. These in turn lead to a desire for stimulants, the subject of the next chapter, then for relaxants such as alcohol, then to stimulants such as coffee. The result is a never-ending cycle of stress – but natural relaxants can help you break it.

Herbs versus pharmaceuticals

Most of our pharmaceutical drugs are made from plants, or are manufactured copies, modified and refined for more specific actions. The whole herb, on the other hand, is less likely to simply treat symptoms, and more likely to promote the body's natural functions.

Herbs are most effective when used as close to their natural form as possible. This includes using whole extracts rather than isolated 'active ingredients', which is the pharmaceutical model. There are extracts of herbs, standardised for the so-called active ingredients, but standardisation is not a simple matter because herbs are made up of a variety of compounds which work together synergistically. In fact, one of the most remarkable aspects of herbs is that they combine several different healing properties which may act simultaneously on different systems of the body.

Scientific research has revealed that the whole plant is often more effective than any isolated ingredient. When we separate out the active ingredient, we may be losing a significant portion of the plant's action. A case in point is kava. Studies of this plant repeatedly find that the best effects are derived from a whole extract, containing not only a combination of the active fat-soluble compounds kavalactones, but also other supporting factors that are yet to be studied. The same is true for St John's wort. Hypericin, long believed to be the active antidepressant ingredient, has been recently upstaged by hyperforin. The whole plant extract may work better than either of the isolated compounds, indicating an internal synergy. Lastly, concentrating a substance often removes its protective compounds, thus increasing the possibility of side effects, as is the case with the herb ephedra, discussed in Chapter 5.

In Germany, where doctors can prescribe herbal as well as synthetic products, they frequently choose the more benign, and equally effective, herbs.

The most popular and effective natural relaxants are the herbs:

▶ Kava
▶ Valerian
▶ Hops
▶ Passion flower

and the amino acids:

▶ GABA
▶ Taurine

Let's explore how these work and why they are both effective and much better for you than alcohol, cannabis or tranquillisers.

Kava: a Pacific herb

Kava or *Piper methysticum*, which means 'intoxicating pepper', has been consumed as a social and ceremonial drink by Pacific Islanders for over 3,000 years. The first description of this tall, lush plant with heart-shaped leaves came to the West from Captain Cook, on his celebrated voyages through the South Seas. To this day, when village elders or others come together for significant meetings, they begin with an elaborate kava ceremony. It is also used to welcome visiting dignitaries. Pope Paul, Queen Elizabeth II and President Lyndon Johnson have all tried it. Kava is also drunk in less formal social settings as a mild inebriant, like alcohol, often after work.

The root is used both for the drink and, dried, to make the supplements available in the West. Currently, kava is used in Europe and increasingly in the US to counteract stress, anxiety and insomnia. But kava is turning out to be a remarkable substance, also increasingly popular, as in the South

Pacific, as a natural high connector. We will cover that aspect in Chapter 8, 'Connectors'.

Research shows that kava works just as well as well as benzodiazepines.[3] Unlike these prescription drugs, however, you don't need to keep increasing the dose to get the same effect, there are no withdrawal problems when you stop taking it, and a low daytime dose will relax you without making you sleepy. In fact, kava can actually enhance concentration. Research shows that on a word recognition test, it improves reaction time and performance.[4] This makes it easy to use for specific anxiety-producing situations such as a job interview or a final exam, where you want to be both calm and alert. In fact, I (Hyla) use kava tincture when meeting a deadline: it relaxes my mind and body and cuts out mental chatter, while keeping me alert and focused.

In higher doses, kava is a natural sleep enhancer. Unlike benzodiazepines, though, it does not suppress REM (rapid eye movement, which occurs during dreaming) sleep, essential to our emotional, mental and physical well-being. And there's no morning hangover, either.

Why kava is better than alcohol

Like alcohol, kava can help you relax and ease social interactions. But of the two only kava allows you to maintain a clear mind, with no hangover. As novelist and travel writer Paul Theroux says in *The Happy Isles of Oceania*:

> No one ever went haywire and beat up his wife after bingeing on yanggona [kava]. No one ever staggered home from a night around the kava bowl and thrashed his children, or insulted his boss, or got tattooed, or committed rape. The usual effect after a giggly interval was the staggers and then complete paralysis.

After the first 2 hours of use, alcohol can make you nervous and shaky. Kava, on the other hand, is calming. One 4-week German study of patients diagnosed with anxiety found that participants experienced dramatic improvements in anxiety symptoms after just 1 week of kava use, with improvement continuing through week 4. In the largest (101 participants) and longest (25 weeks) study to date, by Dr H. P. Volz in Germany, kava provided significant relief of anxiety versus the placebo, or 'dummy' pill, and with minimal side-effects.[5]

How kava works

Kava acts both on the limbic system, the emotional centre of the brain, and directly on muscles, so it actually promotes relaxation in two different ways. The muscle-relaxing effects make it particularly useful in treating headaches, backaches and other tension-related pain.

The active ingredients, as we've seen, are kavalactones, taken from the powdered lateral roots of the plant. As they are fat or lipid soluble, and don't dissolve in water, they form an emulsion or oil and water mixture in the traditional drink. Kava is selectively cultivated for specific effects: certain combinations of these cultivars are more relaxing, others more stimulating, and still others more intoxicating. Those cultivars prized for their ability to alter consciousness in various ways are generally kept for island use while the rest are exported, much as vintners will hold on to their prized vintages.

Kava's specific effect on neurotransmitters is not entirely clear. It appears, though, that, in keeping with its relaxant effects, it enhances the receptivity of the brain's GABA receptors. Unlike alcohol, though, it neither disturbs blood sugar balance, nor reduces endorphin levels.

How much should you take? Kava is available in various forms – tablets, capsules and tinctures, and even in sprays. The taste is quite strong, so most people prefer tablets or capsules to the liquid. The recommended daily adult dose is 60 to 75mg of kavalactones, taken two to three times daily. This is equivalent to 200 to 250mg of standardised extract containing 30 per cent kavalactones, or 100 to 150mg of 55 per cent extract or 100mg of 75 per cent extract. As a sedative to aid sleep, the dose is two to three times that amount. For getting high and chilling out, the dose is quite individual, generally two to three times the dose used to help you sleep.

All these numbers may be confusing, but remember, herbs are extracted from natural plants, not manufactured, and the markers such as kavalactones in this case are given as a percentage of the whole extract. Conveniently, most capsules or tablets are in the range of 60 to 75mg of kavalactones each. Then, your dose is an individual matter, depending on your own chemistry. Don't be too concerned with the exact numbers. Rather, start with one capsule and observe your response. Then you can adjust accordingly. The first time or two some people feel a little groggy, so just in case, start on a weekend or evening when you don't have to be fully alert. After a few doses, your body gets used to the feel, and you will probably feel relaxed, but alert. Of course, if you are using it to zone out, just let it happen.

The tinctures are an acquired taste. They are rather bitter, and will numb the inside of your mouth for a few minutes. An advantage to this form is the rapid onset. Taken straight, it is rapidly absorbed in the mouth and so into the bloodstream even before you swallow. If you prefer, you can take the tincture in fruit juice to cover the taste.

Side-effects

Taken in these typical doses, kava has no known side-effects except for occasional skin rashes in sensitive individuals, headache or mild stomach upset. Chronic high dose use on the islands (say, 20 times the recommended daily dose every day for 10 years) can lead to a scaly yellow skin rash called 'kava dermopathy'. This eventually disappears when use of the herb is stopped.

A word of caution: kava should not be taken with alcohol or other sedatives because of its additive effect. You should never drive after using it in higher doses. Because high doses of kava can cause intoxication, there is concern that it could become a herb of abuse. There have already been a few arrests for erratic driving under the influence, which only serves to give this natural relaxant a bad name.

There have also been media reports of young people trying to get high by taking products they thought contained kava. Exploiting its exotic appeal, bottles of a product called 'fX' were distributed at a Los Angeles

New Year's Eve celebration, and promoted as kava. There were hundreds of adverse reactions, widely reported in the press as due to kava. Unfortunately, less attention was paid some time later when the police report revealed that fX did contain dangerous drugs – but no kava at all.

For information on using kava to help in quitting tranquillisers, see the Appendix, page 286. For more details on kava see Hyla's book *Kava: Nature's Answer to Stress, Anxiety and Insomnia.*

Kava

How it works: Calms the limbic system, the emotional centre of the brain and relaxes muscles, likely through an indirect action on GABA receptors.

Positive effects:
▶ Relaxes mind, emotions and muscles, making it useful for headaches, backaches and other tension
▶ Reduces excessive mental chatter
▶ Increases mental focus
▶ Expands our overall awareness
▶ No habituation, tolerance, addiction or hangover.

Cautions: Do not drive or operate heavy machinery after use. Do not mix with alcohol, as the two substances seem to potentiate each other. Do not take while using benzodiazepines.

How much?: As a relaxant, the normal dosage is approximately 60–75mg of kavalactones. As a bedtime sedative, 120–200mg.

Valerian: nature's Valium

Another favourite for the treatment of anxiety is valerian (*Valeriana officinalis*), sometimes referred to as 'nature's Valium'. Derived from the dried rhizomes and roots of this tall plant, which grows on wet soil in many countries, it has been used for thousands of years as a folk remedy. As a natural relaxant it is useful for several disorders including restlessness, nervousness, insomnia, menstrual problems and 'nervous' stomach. Like the Valium-type drugs, valerian acts on the brain's GABA receptors, offering a similar tranquillising action without the same side-effects.

Be forewarned, though – its smell has been likened to old socks! So hold your nose, and here's how to take it. Using standardised extract (0.8 per cent valeric acid), the dose is 50 to 100mg, two to three times daily for relaxation. For bedtime sedation to promote sleep, take 150 to 300mg about 45 minutes before bedtime.

Another word of caution: valerian can interact with alcohol, as well as with certain antihistamines, muscle relaxants, psychotropic drugs and narcotics. Those taking any of these drugs should take valerian only under the supervision of a healthcare practitioner.

For information on using valerian to help in quitting tranquillisers, see the Appendix, page 286.

Valerian

How it works: Enhances GABA activity.

Positive effects: Reduces anxiety, insomnia, tension.

Cautions: Potentiates sedative drugs, including muscle relaxants and antihistamines. Can interact with alcohol.

How much?: As a relaxant: 50–100mg twice a day. As a bedtime sedative: 150–300mg about 45 minutes before bedtime.

The next two herbs are long-time sedating herbs that you will often find in combination formulas. Like many subtle flavourings, however, they do add their own special qualities to the mix, and you might like to know something about them.

Hops: happy snoozing

Hops (*Humulus lupulus*) have been used for centuries as a mild sedative and sleeping aid. The herb's primary use is to calm nerves and induce sleep, usually in combination with other herbal sedatives such as passion flower, valerian and skullcap. Its sedative action works directly on the central nervous system. The dose is around 200mg per day, but varies from formula to formula.

Passion flower: rest easy

The mild sedative effect of passion flower (*Passiflora incarnata*) has been well substantiated in numerous animal and human studies. The herb encourages deep, restful, uninterrupted sleep, with no side-effects. Passion flower has been commonly used in the treatment of concentration problems in schoolchildren and as a sedative for the elderly. In high doses, passion flower has been found to be mildly hallucinogenic, though we don't recommend trying it for that. Dosage varies with the formula, but is generally 100 to 200mg per day of the standardised product.

Relaxing Naturally 2: Amino Acids

GABA: truly chilled

We've now heard quite a lot about GABA, the main inhibitory or calming amino acid/neurotransmitter. GABA regulates the neurotransmitters noradrenalin, dopamine and serotonin, making it a significant mood modulator in both directions. That is, it helps shift a tense, worried state to relaxation, and a blue mood to a happy one. When your levels of GABA are low, you feel anxious, tense, depressed and have trouble sleeping.[6] When your levels increase, your breathing and heart rate slow down and your muscles relax. So it's a welcome addition to any chill-out programme.

While you can enhance GABA activity with herbs, as we've seen, you can also take GABA directly in powder or pill form – 1000mg twice daily after meals. A review article on GABA by two psychiatrists, I. S. Shiah and N. Yatham, at the University of British Columbia in Vancouver, makes it clear that it is able to move easily from the bloodstream into the brain.[7] In technical terms, this crossing of the blood-brain barrier is often an obstacle to a product's effectiveness.

GABA

How it works: Acts directly on the brain as a calming, mood-enhancing neurotransmitter.

Positive effects: Reduces anxiety, insomnia and tension.

Cautions: Can cause nausea and vomiting at high doses.

How much?: 500–1000mg twice daily after meals.

Taurine: calming influence

Taurine is an amino acid that plays a major role in the brain as an 'inhibitory' neurotransmitter. Similar in structure and function to GABA, it provides a similar anti-anxiety effect by helping to calm or stabilise an excited brain. It has many other uses as well, in treating migraine, insomnia, agitation, restlessness, irritability, alcoholism, obsessions, depression and even hypomania/mania – the 'high' phase of bipolar disorder or manic depression.

By inhibiting the release of adrenalin, taurine also protects us from anxiety and other adverse effects of stress. It even helps control high blood pressure.

Since taurine is highly concentrated in animal and fish protein or organ meats, vegetarians can be at risk of taurine deficiency. Taurine is a non-essential amino acid, so our body can manufacture it in the liver and brain from the amino acids L-cysteine and L-methionine if supplied with the required co-factor, vitamin B6. The dose is usually 500 to 1000mg twice daily, and higher as needed.

Taurine

How it works: Enhances GABA activity.

Positive effects: Reduces anxiety, irritability, insomnia, migraine, alcoholism, obsessions and depression.

Cautions: None reported.

How much?: 500–1000mg twice daily.

Action Plan for Natural Relaxation

Getting and staying relaxed will mean making changes. See Part 3 for ways to alter your lifestyle. Changing your chemistry is just as vital. Here's how you do it.

1. Balance your blood sugar: an even keel

There are three golden rules for keeping your blood sugar levels even:

▷ Avoid, or at least considerably reduce, all sugar and stimulants (see Chapter 5 for natural alternatives).

▷ Eat regularly and eat low-GI foods that keep your blood sugar level even.

▷ Supplement the 'energy nutrients', primarily B vitamins and vitamin C, which help to turn your food efficiently into energy.

All these are explained in Chapter 3, 'Natural High Basics'. If you are very stressed, or suspect you have a blood sugar problem, you will also benefit from adding 200mcg of chromium, a mineral that helps insulin to keep your blood sugar level stable, in the morning.

2. Mobilise GABA: the big chill-out

The following herbs and amino acids help to calm down the stress response and act as natural relaxants. The ideal daily doses of all of them are less when combined than when a substance is taken alone.

Natural Relaxant	Combined	Alone
Kava	100mg	200mg*
Valerian	50mg	300mg
Hops	100mg	200mg
Passion flower	100mg	200mg
GABA	500mg	1000mg
Taurine	500mg	1000mg

* The kava dosage given here relates to the actual amount of kavalactones in the product, be it powder, capsules or tincture. Also experiment with kava on its own, in increments of 60–75mg.

3. Take the following to chill out

▶ A good all-round multivitamin supplying optimal amounts of B vitamins, vitamin C (see 'Natural High Basics', Chapter 3) with an optional 200mcg of chromium.

▶ A 'chill-out' formula providing kava, valerian, hops, passion flower, GABA and taurine, as needed.

▶ For a good night's sleep, take 150 to 300mg of valerian and 120 to 180mg of kava about 45 minutes before bedtime, plus 200mg of 5-HTP (see page 173). We recommend starting one new product at a time, observing your response, then adding in a new one as needed. Or take each one on its own for a few days before beginning to combine them.

For a full natural chill-out programme, see 'Top Tips' in Part 4.

STIMULANTS

BURSTING WITH energy, cheerful, wide-awake – we all want that buzz. We can get more done, and done well, when we're feeling alive and alert. It means we can stay the course, and keep up the pace.

But it's some pace these days. As we'll see, in the twenty-first century everyone seems to be travelling in the fast lane. And it's all perhaps a bit overstimulating in other ways, with coffee shops beckoning on every corner and sugar fixes cramming the supermarket shelves. How did it happen?

To a large extent we find the roots of our own need for stimulants in the Industrial Revolution. It demanded brutally long hours from workers and complete exhaustion was an ever-present possibility. Factory owners fuelled them with tea, coffee and tobacco, as a means of pushing them to work faster and more efficiently. Soon sugar joined the mix to sweeten the drinks and finally, chocolate. Ever-increasing consumption continued right up into the twentieth century and rapidly became part of the daily rituals of people throughout Europe. It continues to grow in the new millennium.

These 'workers' friends' aren't the only stimulants around, of course. Amphetamines, cocaine and even alcohol – both a stimulant and relaxant – fall into this category too. All of them affect the emotional centre of the brain, the limbic system, and the stimulating neurotransmitter dopamine, which works together with serotonin, GABA and the endorphins to produce that cherished experience of pleasure. (Chapter 3 delved into this territory, too.) But aside from issues of illegality or serious health consequences, those popular stimulants, in the end, just add to our load of exhaustion.

We'll be looking at the wellsprings of that exhaustion and the substances that offer a quick-fix solution – which ultimately turns into part of the problem. And we'll see how ancient herbs and natural nutrients can give us back our buzz.

The Exhaustion Epidemic

Our own Technological Revolution has spawned a world that never sleeps. Television, the Internet and even the stock market call to us 24 hours a day, 7 days a week. When we shave an hour off our sleep, we feel we've gained some small advantage.

Many of us are also trying to keep impossible schedules of work and family responsibilities. And it has a cumulative effect. You struggle to find time with your kids, friends and colleagues, not to mention your partner. You're less alert than you'd like, feeling drowsy as the day wears on, dozing off if you sit down to read or watch TV in the evening. When you finally do get together with your partner at bedtime, neither of you has energy for anything more than falling asleep.

Too often today we rely on chemical 'helpers' to keep us going: the frequent coffee breaks, the doughnut to satisfy our hunger when we have no time to eat, the cigarette to calm our nerves. You will soon see why we use stimulants, how the common stimulants affect us, how we become dependent on them, and how to replace them with healthier, more effective alternatives.

Energy Check

To get an idea of how depleted your energy might be and how dependent you are on stimulants, check yourself out in the following questionnaire.

Score 1 for each 'yes' answer.

How Tired Are You?	Yes	No
Do you have trouble getting up in the morning?	☐	☐
Do you rely on a cup of coffee to get you going in the morning?	☐	☐
Do you feel tired all the time?	☐	☐
Do you often feel foggy, fuzzy or dull?	☐	☐
Do you have trouble concentrating?	☐	☐

Do you use sugar, caffeine (tea, coffee, caffeinated cola drinks) or a cigarette as a pick-me-up throughout the day?	☐	☐
Are you often irritable or angry, for no apparent reason?	☐	☐
Do your moods seem to go up and down for no apparent reason?	☐	☐
Are your mood swings often relieved by food, especially sweets?	☐	☐
Do you have trouble falling asleep at night?	☐	☐
Do you have headaches or shaky feelings that are relieved by sugar, caffeine or cigarettes?	☐	☐
Do you suspect you're addicted to coffee, caffeinated cola or cigarettes?	☐	☐
Do you find yourself operating from crisis to crisis?	☐	☐
Are you drawn to thrills, danger and drama in your life?	☐	☐

If your score is:

Below 5: You're doing fine. We all have our moments – bad moods, feeling tired or foggy, and in need of a pick-me-up.

5 to 10: You are showing signs of an over-dependence on stimulants to keep you going. This next section will explain what is happening in your body, and how to make healthier choices.

More than 10: You are seriously hooked on stimulants, and it is affecting your mental and physical health. It's important for you to take yourself off them. We will show you how, both in the following pages and in the Appendix, page 279.

What's Up with Stimulants?

An Addicted Society

An extreme of stimulant-seeking behaviour is the problem of addiction. In the US alone, there are 6 million cocaine addicts, 25 million people addicted to nicotine and 14.9 million people who abuse other substances. Of concern, too, are the large numbers of school and university students experimenting with these substances. There are also about 54 million people who are at least 20 per cent overweight – food addicts – and 448,000 compulsive gamblers.

If you give in to your cravings for stimulants, it does not necessarily mean you are weak or 'bad', but simply that your chemistry is controlling you. You need the right fuel – foods, vitamins and other micronutrients – to run your body's engine. (See Chapter 3, 'Natural High Basics'.) You also need sufficient sleep to restore body and mind, and maintain your energy level.

You might even have a chronic viral infection, or an imbalance in your hormones, such as an underactive thyroid gland, that make you tired. In any case turning to stimulants to get your engine going further depletes your already bankrupt system.

The reason why they work in the short term, and the reason why they don't in the long term, is that stimulants affect your blood sugar levels. As we saw in the last chapter stress, sugar and stimulants all raise your blood sugar, which can give you a short-term boost in energy. But, in time, your blood sugar level becomes more and more unstable. (One of the reasons for this is that the body becomes less and less sensitive to the hormone insulin because the insulin receptors have downregulated.) So now you need more stimulants to keep you going. Eventually you become dependent on stimulants. It's a vicious cycle of stress, over-use of stimulants and fatigue. The end result is addiction – and exhaustion.

Addiction can also have genetic or social roots. Often, for instance, addictions run in families. Programmed in your genes, you may be hard-wired for stimulant addiction. Termed Reward Deficiency Syndrome (RDS) by researcher Kenneth Blum, a deficiency in the dopamine receptors can lead to a greater and greater need for stimulation, and ultimately alcohol and stimulant addiction. Remember, when these receptors are stimulated, we feel energised, motivated and happy. A relative lack of these receptors, on the other hand, leads to the opposite – depression, low self-esteem, low energy, a lack of motivation and irritability. RDS is a predisposition only: you are not a slave to your genes. There are ways to deal with the problem, as we will see.

We can also learn addictive behaviour from our families as we're growing up. Joan's parents, for example, would give her chocolate as a treat or reward on special occasions. Since it reminds her of the simple pleasures of childhood, she still comforts herself with hot chocolate or a chocolate bar when times get rough. Many children are raised on sugary

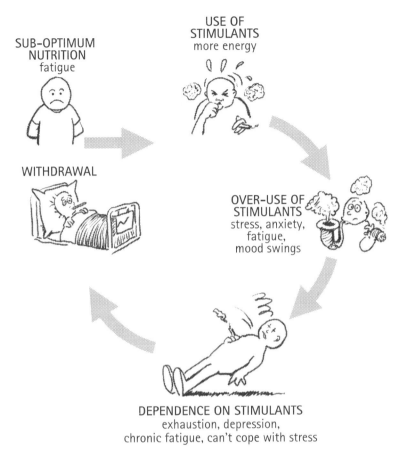

SUB-OPTIMUM
NUTRITION
fatigue

USE OF
STIMULANTS
more energy

WITHDRAWAL

OVER-USE OF
STIMULANTS
stress, anxiety,
fatigue,
mood swings

DEPENDENCE ON STIMULANTS
exhaustion, depression,
chronic fatigue, can't cope with stress

The vicious cycle of stress, stimulants, dependence and fatigue

cereals, caffeine and sugar-laden fizzy drinks, leaving them hooked. Jerry's is another case in point: his teenage friends smoked cigarettes, so he joined them to fit in and look cool. At 40, he is an addicted smoker.

As for the illegal stimulants such as amphetamines and cocaine, users inevitably find it increasingly difficult to relax while living on them. They then use relaxants such as alcohol, sleeping pills, tranquillisers and marijuana to bring them down. It's an addictive cycle that impairs performance, promotes stress and depletes energy.

Handle with Care: Popular Stimulants

Stimulants have been around the block a few times. Since prehistory, people have used a variety of substances to motivate, energise and inspire. Native North Americans smoke tobacco, the natives of the Andes chew coca leaves, the Indians and Chinese drink tea. And then there are our Western offerings: sugar, tea, coffee, cigarettes, stimulant drugs. In this section we will explore the effects of these substances, including others containing caffeine, such as chocolate, guarana, mate and kola nut. We'll also look at ephedra or ma huang and yohimbe.

Popular they may be, but as we've seen they're also problematic. As you can see from the diagram opposite, all stimulants work by mimicking or triggering the release of the three neurotransmitters dopamine, adrenalin and noradrenalin. That's what makes you feel motivated and high. We learned earlier how downregulation in the brain eventually puts a stop to the fun of getting high. That's exactly what happens with stimulants. This over-stimulation leads to downregulation, where the receptor sites for dopamine, adrenalin and noradrenalin start to shut down. You keep needing more of the product to feel the same effect. But how much is too much, and are there some stimulants we can take safely in moderation?

While a substance can be good in one context, it can be harmful in another. In one short-term experiment, coffee was shown to heighten alertness, but those studies are not looking at memory impairment or increased blood pressure in habitual coffee drinkers.[1] Also, researchers are not always without bias, and may interpret results to fit their preconceptions or desired outcome.

We'll deal with these issues as we discuss each substance in detail. But for now let us say some stimulants are never recommended, while others can be acceptable (in moderation) depending on the situation.

Sugar: toxic treat

Sugar is a fairly recent entry into the stimulant game. Of course, it's always been available in natural sources such as fruit, with its slow-releasing fructose and fibre. Refined sugar, however, only came in with the Industrial

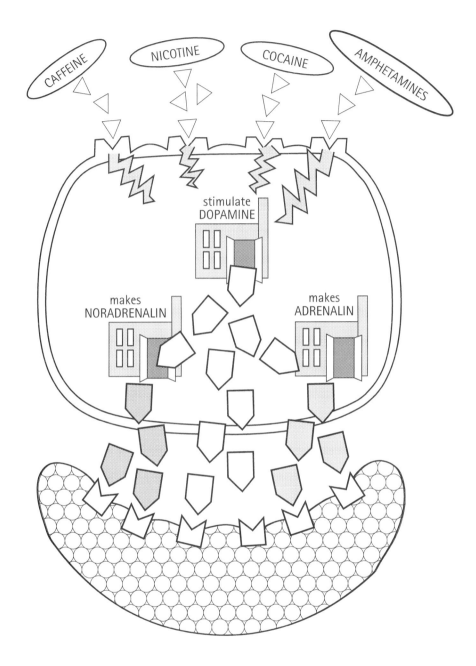

The stimulants release the three neurotransmitters, which then raise blood sugar levels

Revolution; yet today, we can hardly picture a celebration without sweet treats – birthday and wedding cakes, Christmas puddings, Easter chocolates.

How can such a delicious, seemingly harmless children's treat be so damaging? Rapidly absorbed and broken down quickly into molecules of glucose, it quickly reaches the brain, producing feelings of 'comfort' or 'energy'. Sugar bingeing looks a lot like any other addiction – tolerance develops, and you need more to get the same effect. How serious is that?

Downside of Sugar

Sugar is bad for you.

▶ While a valuable fuel for our cells, it can be toxic when consumed in excess, often causing damage to the arteries, kidneys, eyes and nerves.

▶ The body tries to get it out of the blood as quickly as possible, but this can then cause a 'rebound' low blood sugar with its own set of problems. Some people feel stimulated immediately after taking it, then become cranky and finally go into a low blood sugar slump.

Caffeine: brewing up trouble

Found in over a hundred plants throughout the world, caffeine is consumed primarily in beverages. A half-dozen caffeine-containing plants are more widely used than all other herbal materials combined!

Over a thousand years ago, Muslims used coffee for religious rituals. When the stuff finally reached Europe in the seventeenth century, it was seen by the authorities as a dangerous drug. Nonetheless, coffeehouses spread, as did dependence on this new drug. The rest is history. Together with tea, it comprises 97 per cent of worldwide caffeine consumption. Some parts of the world use other forms of caffeine – mate, guarana and kola nut – which are now becoming more popular in the West.

Caffeine was first isolated from coffee in 1821. The effects of coffee are more potent than those of caffeine alone since it contains two other stimulants – theophylline and theobromine. These weaker versions of caffeine are also found in decaffeinated coffee. All three are xanthines, alkaloid compounds that occur in both plants and animals.

The main reason people drink coffee is that its caffeine content boosts mood and energy. It does this by blocking the receptors for a brain chemical called *adenosine*, whose function is to stop dopamine release. With less adenosine activity, then, you increase dopamine and adrenalin. You then feel alert, motivated and stimulated, though some people will feel uncomfortable and jittery. In 30 to 60 minutes, caffeine reaches its peak concentration. It is then inactivated by the liver, with only half its peak level left after 4 to 6 hours.

So where's the danger? Caffeine is highly addictive. Research shows that consuming as little as 100mg a day can lead to withdrawal symptoms when you stop, including headache, fatigue, difficulty concentrating and drowsiness. It's worth knowing that while a small cup of instant coffee may contain less than 100mg of caffeine, a large 'designer' coffee can contain as much as 500mg – five times the 'addictive' dose. Even more chemicals are used in manufacturing decaffeinated coffee, and in the end it still contains traces of caffeine – about 0.3mg per 140ml or 5fl oz cup.

Downside of Caffeine

▶ Overstimulation of the central nervous system, leading to: increased risk of heart attacks, irritability, insomnia and rapid and irregular heartbeats.

▶ Elevated blood sugar and cholesterol levels.

▶ Heartburn and other gastrointestinal problems.

▶ Fibrocystic breast disease.

▶ Diuresis (excessive urination) which can lead to dehydration.

> ▶ Used during pregnancy, it increases the risk of birth defects.
>
> ▶ Contains tars, phenols and other carcinogens.
>
> ▶ Pesticides are used in growing the coffee beans.
>
> ▶ Toxic chemicals are used to extract it.

At best, we can say that coffee has minor short-term mental and emotional benefits, but these are not sustained. A study published in the *American Journal of Psychiatry* observed 1,500 psychology students divided into four categories depending on their coffee intake: abstainers, low consumers (1 cup or equivalent a day), moderate (1 to 5 cups a day) and high (5 or more cups a day). On psychological testing, the moderate and high consumers had higher levels of anxiety and depression than the abstainers, and the high consumers had a higher incidence of stress-related medical problems coupled with lower academic performance.[2]

The bottom line? Use in moderation, if not complete abstinence.

Tea: not so refreshing

Tea (*Camellia sinensis*) has been a favourite stimulant in many countries for centuries. Black tea is prepared by an initial slow drying of the fresh leaves, which allows them to begin to ferment, while for green tea, the leaves are dried quickly. Both contain caffeine.

The drinking of tea began in ancient Asia, and eventually the beverage became Britain's standard 'refresher'. Introduced in the seventeenth century, by the early nineteenth century it had become a highly sought-after stimulant for the newly industrialising society, providing energy to goad the workers into faster production. And as it required lots of sugar to enhance its bitter taste, it gave the economy another boost from sugar sales.

The cuppa continues to be a significant pick-me-up and social ritual in Britain, where tea consumption is four times that of coffee. In the US the figures are reversed. You can guess why by recalling the historic Boston

Tea Party, which preceded the American Revolution. Rather than pay a tea tax to their oppressors across the sea, the colonists dumped boxes of imported tea from British trade ships into the harbour – and haven't had much taste for it since.

Tea's stimulating effects come from caffeine, theobromine and theophylline, the same compounds as in coffee. Because of different methods of preparation and the many varieties of the cultivated plant, the average caffeine content of tea ranges widely from about 1 per cent to over 4 per cent. The box below lists the downsides of drinking tea (and see also the coffee downsides on page 75). Green tea, however, does have some redeeming features. It's discussed on page 101.

Downside of Tea

▶ A strong cup of tea contains as much caffeine as a weak cup of coffee – with all the attendant risks (see box, pages 75–6).

▶ Tannin content interferes with absorption of minerals.

Colas: message in a bottle

Cola drinks contain about a half to a quarter of the caffeine found in a weak cup of coffee. The original Coca-Cola even contained small amounts of coca (cocaine), hence the name. Today's drinks usually contain sugar and colourings, which also act as stimulants. Maybe worse, diet drinks contain the artificial sweetener aspartame (Nutrasweet) which can be toxically overstimulating to the brain. We have seen people who thought they were 'going crazy' with anxiety, insomnia and disordered thinking magically recover when they stopped their diet drinks. Ironically, although touted as a diet product, they can actually cause weight gain. (See http://www.dorway.com/blayenn.html for scientific information on this chemical, and Resources on page 304.)

More recently, new soft drinks have been introduced that push up the levels of caffeine they contain, boosting both their kick and addictiveness.

Shades of the tobacco industry! With such names as Jolt or Red Bull, their caffeine content can equal or even surpass that of a cup of coffee. Children and young people are drinking large amounts of them, especially relative to their weight, thereby exposing their developing brains and bodies to a hazardous substance. Never mind illicit drugs – junk food and caffeinated drinks bought by parents can lead to serious health problems and addictions in children.

Downside of Colas

► Contain caffeine – with all the attendant risks (see box, pages 75–6).

► Sugar and colouring are added stimulants, while aspartame in diet versions can toxically overstimulate the brain.

► New drinks aimed at young people have even higher levels of caffeine.

Some medications for the relief of headaches, such as Anadin, contain caffeine. Other caffeine tablets such as Pro Plus and the herb guarana (see page 80) are sold outright as stimulants.

CAFFEINE BUZZOMETER

Product	Caffeine content
Coca-Cola Classic 350ml (12 fl oz)	46mg
Diet Coke 350ml (12 fl oz)	46mg
Red Bull 250ml (9 fl oz)	90mg
Hot cocoa 150ml (5 fl oz)	10mg
Coffee, instant 150ml (5 fl oz)	40–105mg
Coffee, espresso, cappuccino, latte	30–50mg
Coffee, filter 150ml (5 fl oz)	110–150mg
Coffee, Starbucks (grande)	500mg
Decaffeinated coffee 150ml (5 fl oz)	0.3mg
Tea 150ml (5 fl oz)	20–100mg

Chocolate cake (1 slice)	20–30mg
Bittersweet chocolate 28g (1 oz)	5–35mg
Pro Plus	50mg
PEP	30mg

Death by chocolate?

Chocolate's major active ingredient is cocoa, a significant source of the stimulant theobromine. Research by British psychologist, Dr David Benton at the University of Wales in Swansea, showed chocolate to be an excellent mood elevator. When he played sad music to a group of students, their mood sank. He then offered them the choice of milk chocolate or carob, a natural chocolate substitute that was similar in taste. Without their knowing which product they were eating, the participants found that the chocolate raised their mood, while the carob didn't. Moreover, as their mood fell, their cravings for chocolate increased.[3]

In addition to theobromine – as we've seen, also found in tea and coffee – chocolate also contains the mood-enhancing stimulant, phenethylamine. Both of these stimulate dopamine production. Even laboratory rats with an alcohol addiction, when given the choice, will replace some of their alcohol intake with chocolate.

A recent study of mice and rats shows that dopamine kick-starts a brain messenger chemical called DARP-32 that in turn activates hormones that make females more interested in sex.[4] Without even knowing about DARP-32, generations of lonely, frustrated men and women have binged on chocolate, with sometimes surprising results. Valentine's Day chocolates say it all.

The bad news? Too much chocolate, especially the highly sweetened kind, causes all the problems of going overboard on sugar, including weight gain. It is often high in fats too. The addictive nature of it suggests the development of tolerance, such as 'just one chocolate' will no longer do. It becomes, instead, 'just one *more*'. In addition, like coffee, cocoa beans are grown in countries where pesticide use is unregulated, exposing the consumer to cancer-causing compounds.

If you are going to eat chocolate, eat the pure, dark, preferably organic stuff, not cheap bars full of fat and sugar. But, as with any stimulant, if you eat it every day, or find yourself craving it, you've gone too far. Keep chocolate as a special treat, not a daily ritual.

Downside of Chocolate

► Contains caffeine – with all the attendant risks (see box, page 75).

► Often high in sugar and fats, leading to weight gain.

► Can be treated with carcinogenic pesticides in country of origin.

Guarana, mate, kola nut: caffeine by any other name

The name guarana conjures up exotic images of tribal people in the Amazonian rainforests, living in harmony with nature. And if it's 'natural' it must be good for you. Right? Well, not exactly. The seeds and leaves of the guarana plant, a climbing shrub native to Brazil and Uruguay, are high in caffeine.

A traditional social drink, appetite suppressant and aphrodisiac, guarana is used extensively in South America today in soft drinks. Because it contains saponins, compounds found in ginseng, there are tonic or balancing properties in these native preparations (see page 88). They also have a mild and long-lasting effect, and are less irritating to the gastrointestinal tract than, say, coffee. This is probably due to the presence of fats and oils in the seeds, which prolong absorption. Most commercially prepared products, on the other hand, are absorbed and used up in the body as quickly as a cup of coffee. Once more, the closer we stick to the natural forms of a product, the healthier it is for us.

A dried paste made chiefly from the crushed seed of guarana has a relatively high caffeine content, ranging from 2.5 to 5 per cent and averaging about 3.5 per cent. To determine how much caffeine there is in any product, you must again do your maths. You can multiply the total weight of the capsule or powder by the percentage of caffeine or guarana to get the number of milligrams of caffeine per dose.

The conclusion regarding its use? Like tea or coffee, it can be over-stimulating, and have the same ill effects. In a dilute, milder form, it can be used as an occasional pick-me-up for those whose adrenal status is healthy – that is, not suffering from stress or burnout.

Another traditional South American stimulant is the jungle tea mate (pronounced 'matay'). The dried leaves of this low-growing bush are brewed into a hot drink. Besides low concentrations of caffeine, mate contains theophylline (0.05 per cent), theobromine (0.1 to 2 per cent), tannins, vitamins and minerals. At 15 to 25mg of caffeine per cup, as in green tea, mate is used for enhancing alertness and concentration. It can be useful on occasion, but as with any stimulant, excessive use can tax the adrenal glands.

Kola nut is used as an aphrodisiac, probably working in the same way as chocolate. The nut (*Cola nitida*) is a seed kernel related to the cacao tree, and is native to the rainforests of West Africa. It is also cultivated in the West Indies and other tropical areas. Containing up to 3 per cent caffeine, its stimulant properties were originally derived from chewing on the seeds. It is now available as tea made of ground seeds. Kola nut was the 'cola' part of Coke which, as we mentioned earlier, originally also contained coca extract. Cola drinks now get their kick from synthesised or extracted caffeine plus sugar.

Downsides of Guarana, Mate and Kola Nut

► All contain caffeine – with all the attendant risks (see box, page 75).

► Guarana and mate can only be used by those with healthy adrenal status – not the seriously stressed.

Ephedra (ma huang): life in the fast lane

Though a traditional remedy with a long history of use, ephedra has become a controversial herb – within both the natural products industry and government regulatory agencies – because of the way some people use it now. Called ma huang (*Ephedra sinica*), this ancient Chinese remedy triggers the release of adrenalin, the hormone that mediates the stress response. Since the stress response also causes an initial surge in energy, as well as suppression of appetite, ephedra is often used for both quick energy and weight loss. One study found that it worked better than Redux, a weight loss drug that was later withdrawn from the market because of toxic effects. A 1996 study found that a combination of 30mg of ephedra, 100mg of caffeine and 300mg of aspirin promoted fat-burning.[5] Ephedra is also used as a decongestant, most commonly as ephedrine, a synthetic version of ephedra which is more potent and longer-lasting.

Ephedra is also used by some for recreation. Often advertised as 'herbal Ecstasy', ephedra actually has little in common with the entheogen Ecstasy or MDMA (see chapter 8). Rather, what's marketed as herbal Ecstasy is generally a combination of ephedra and caffeine, both of them in high doses, which causes a 'rush' that is stimulating and energising. The high-dose combination can be dangerous, however, producing a rapid heart rate and a rise in blood pressure with accompanying headache, dizziness and, on rare occasions, even death.

Having the right information will help you make the correct choice of whether or not to use ephedra. It is relatively safe at doses of 15 to 25mg, and for a short period of time – weeks, not months. You should not take it if you are energy-depleted, recovering from any illness or have a weak constitution. Athletes often use it as a stimulant, and while it increases their exercise tolerance, they too should use it only in the short term.

Downsides of Ephedra

▶ Too much can lead to headache, tremor, insomnia and anxiety.

▶ Rapid heart rate, irregular heart rhythm and a rise in blood pressure.

▶ Increased risk of heart attack or stroke in susceptible individuals.

▶ Reversible toxic psychosis from overstimulation of the brain.

▶ A weakened heart, adrenals and other organs in the long term.

CONTRAINDICATIONS:
It should not be taken by:

▶ Pregnant or breast-feeding women.

▶ Children.

▶ In combination with the so-called 'MAOI' antidepressant drugs.

The natural products industry and publications in the US have taken action to educate the public, and to provide quality, safe products. Such organisations include the Ephedra Committee of AHPA, the American Herbal Products Association (www.ahpa.org) and the American Botanical Council (www.herbalgram.org) whose extensive article on the subject can be seen on their website.[6] In the UK, ephedra is a restricted herb that can be prescribed by registered herbalists and pharmacists, but is not available for sale over the counter to members of the public.

Yohimbe: too hot

A traditional African herb, yohimbe is as controversial a stimulant as ephedra. In its extracted alkaloid form, yohimbine, it is used not only as a mood enhancer and weight-loss product, but also as an aphrodisiac. In fact, yohimbine hydrochloride in 5.4mg tablets is prescribed by doctors in the USA to treat impotence.

Yohimbe enhances the stimulant neurotransmitters, dopamine and noradrenalin. As with other stimulants, it affects different people differently. For some, there is a pleasant enhancement of the senses, increase in empathy and communication, and enhanced sexual arousal. Men can have long-lasting erections, and powerful ejaculations. On the other hand, many feel uncomfortably stimulated with rapid heart rate, headache, anxiety and insomnia. Taking yohimbe can also cause a dangerous rise in blood pressure.

The bottom line? It appears safe for occasional use, with the proper precautions. It should not be taken by those who suffer from hypertension.

Downside of Yohimbe

▶ Can cause uncomfortable overstimulation – rapid heart rate, headache, anxiety and insomnia.

▶ Can cause a dangerous rise in blood pressure.

CONTRAINDICATIONS:
It should not be taken by:

▶ People suffering from hypertension.

Definite Nos: From Smoking to Speed

The tobacco high: all puffed out

Together with caffeine and alcohol, nicotine is one of the three most widely used psychoactive drugs in our society. With no redeeming value, 'smoking will continue as the leading cause of preventable, premature mortality for many years to come', according to the US surgeon-general. In 1999, it killed 120,000 people in the UK alone.

Nicotine, the primary stimulant in cigarettes, has a significant effect even in small doses. In fact, it is such a powerful toxin that one cigar contains enough nicotine to kill several people (and not just from the smell)!

If you have ever smoked, can you recall the sensation of your first cigarette? It probably tasted terrible, burned your mouth and lungs (if you even inhaled), and made you nauseated and dizzy. Those are some of its toxic effects in action. A few more smokes, and for most people, your body no longer rebels. In fact you rather like it. In short – you're hooked.

Nicotine has a complex series of actions, both stimulating and relaxing. It is more addictive than heroin – and is often the hardest addiction to break. It stimulates the adrenals to release adrenalin, raising blood pressure and heart rate, and increases gastrointestinal activity. It also acts as a muscle relaxant.

In the brain, nicotine activates the release of dopamine, exhibiting a stimulant effect similar to that of caffeine. It also has a short-term anti-depressant effect, though this is most often followed by a rebound depression. In larger amounts, nicotine acts as a sedative, probably because of its effect on serotonin. People trying to kick the tobacco habit describe the accompanying tension and irritability as 'feeling like you want to jump out of your skin'. They often experience low blood sugar problems, which leads them to overeat and gain weight.

For details on how to stop smoking see the Appendix, page 275.

Cocaine: down with a crash

Cocaine is probably the best-known and most powerful illegal stimulant. It's the active ingredient of the coca plant, and was first isolated in the West around 1860. The father of psychoanalysis, Freud, experimented with the refined powdered drug personally, and described cocaine as 'magical'. While the coca leaf typically contains between 0.1 and 0.9 per cent cocaine, the concentrated coca paste is 60 to 80 per cent pure cocaine. It works by blocking the re-absorption of dopamine, leaving more in the synapse to interact with the receptors. The leaf is safely used by field labourers in the Andes, to maintain energy.

The concentrated drug, however, leads to an intense 'rush', with enhanced mood, sensory awareness, self-confidence and sexual interest. Unfortunately, this is generally followed by a crash into anxiety, depression, irritability and exhaustion. If the vicious cycle of addiction ensues, there is an intense craving for the next hit, and users follow a downhill course into deterioration of physical and mental health – often emerging as severe depression, agitation and even paranoia.

Amphetamines: mother's little uppers

Popularly known as speed, D-amphetamine has been used for years by long-distance truck drivers, students cramming for finals, and harried housewives needing a lift. Like cocaine, amphetamine blocks neurons' re-absorption of the neurotransmitters noradrenalin and dopamine, but it also triggers their release, doubling its potency.

Amphetamines were discovered and commonly prescribed in the 1960s. In contrast with 'happy pills', these were stimulating ones, allowing the users to do more, focus better and feel more energised – until the pill wore off, and they needed another fix. These drugs were later used as diet pills, and as a treatment for attention deficit disorder (ADD). We have seen how women with food cravings, weight problems, depression and even ADD were given the perfect happy pill for their condition – until the prescription ran out.

Doctors in the US thought they were helping these women but actually turned them into addicts. Legislation then became more rigorous, and in the 1980s the number of these prescriptions fell. The 1990s brought a resurgence, with the mushrooming of medical diet centres, dispensing stimulants such as Fen-Phen and Redux, later found to be dangerous and removed from the market. These substances were banned in the UK from the start. Amphetamines continue to be prescribed for children with ADD, as dexedrine and its relative, Ritalin. In fact, children with ADD are often overstimulated by fast-paced television shows and video games, then expected to be calm and focused in the classroom. Their brains may also be undernourished and over-sugared, both of which can lead to attention and learning problems.

Natural Stimulants: A Better Boost

So now we know what to actively avoid on the stimulant front – or just handle with care. But what about mornings, always a bad time for some of us, or those moments when we're really drained? The good news is that there are a number of substances that stimulate without compromising your health.

These safe and natural supplements don't deplete your reserves. Instead they help you:

▶ Sustain energy

▶ Raise your spirits

▶ Optimise your performance

▶ Overcome cravings to addictive stimulants.

They're non-addictive and don't encourage tolerance: the same dose will give you the same response, consistently.

Several groups of products help restore and enhance energy. These are the 'adaptogenic' herbs, amino acids and vitamins.

'Adaptogenic' herbs include licorice, ginseng (Asian, American or Siberian), ashwaganda, reishi mushroom and rhodiola. The amino acids that stimulate include phenylalanine and tyrosine, while stimulating vitamins include pantothenic acid (vitamin B5) and C, which are needed to make adrenalin and cortisol. Finally, two substances – green tea and the coenzyme NADH – are also excellent additions to your anti-exhaustion arsenal.

Taking these substances isn't going to give you the kind of instant jolt you'd expect from coffee or a cigarette, or the intensity of cocaine or amphetamines. On the other hand, they deliver a consistent and more sustainable level of energy, alertness and well-being. Once you feel this good, your desire for stimulants will fall away. (See Appendix, page 279 to speed up the process.)

The more stressful your lifestyle, the more nutrients you need. To complete your programme, add the energising and destressing exercises covered in Part Three, 'Living High Naturally'.

Adaptogens: support your adrenals

Since the adrenal glands are the foundation of natural energy and stimulation, we will start by looking at your level of adrenal health.

Check your score on the stress quiz (see page 40). If your score is above 40, the chances are your adrenal glands are depleted. Use the recommendations in the following section to help to restore their function. Remember, if you are stressed out, don't use stimulants: they can cause further burnout.

While Western medicine tends to ignore adrenal function unless it is at either extreme, traditional Chinese medicine has subtle ways of diagnosing and treating adrenal overuse and burnout. It relies on the principles of balancing of the opposites in the mind, body and spirit. The goal is to restore natural energy flow, using specific herbs called adaptogens. They help the body adapt to a range of stresses, such as heat, cold, exertion, trauma, sleep deprivation, toxic exposure, radiation, infection and psychological stress. They have few, if any, side-effects, are effective in treating a wide variety of illnesses, and help return the body to homeostasis – its natural balance. By supporting and rebuilding the system in this way, adaptogens promote a feeling of increased energy and well-being, with no tolerance, downregulation or addiction.

Ginseng: king of all tonics

In continuous use in China for over 2,000 years, ginseng, called 'the king of all tonics', restores vital energy throughout the entire body, helping to overcome stress and fatigue and recover from weakness and deficiencies. There are actually three different herbs commonly called ginseng: Asian ginseng (*Panax ginseng*), American ginseng (*Panax quinquefolius*) and Siberian ginseng (*Eleutherococcus senticosus*). The latter herb is actually not ginseng at all, but Russian scientists who researched it found that it functions nearly identically.

Asian ginseng is a perennial that grows in northern China, Korea and Russia. In traditional Chinese terms, Asian ginseng is seen as more *yang* or stimulating, than *yin*. It raises body temperature, strengthens digestion and the lungs, and calms the spirit. Its close relative, American ginseng, is cultivated in the US though largely exported to Asia. It is prized there as a *yin* herb – less heating, less stimulating, and more balanced than Asian ginseng.

The active ingredients are called ginsenosides. There are many different ones, each having their specific effects. Most of the modern-day research has been done on the clinical effects of single components. In 1988, a German university professor, E. Ploss, published a summary and analysis of studies on the clinical use of Asian ginseng, followed in 1990 by a review by Professors Sonnenborn and Proppert.[7] All together, these articles surveyed 37 experiments done between 1968 and 1990, on a total of 2,562 cases, with treatments averaging 2 to 3 months. In 13 studies, the individuals showed an improvement in mood, and in 11, improvement in intellectual performance. All showed a near-absence of side-effects.

Ginseng is available as powdered root in capsules or tablets, or as an alcohol-based tincture. The recommended dose is 100 to 200mg daily of a standardised extract containing 4 to 7 per cent ginsenosides.

The Russians have been far ahead of us in their recognition of Siberian ginseng, a valuable, less costly ginseng-like herb. In the 1940s, the Russian scientist who began researching concluded that it was as good as the 'real' ginsengs. Their athletes take it for months before the Olympics. Cosmonauts taking it remain alert and energetic, despite the physical and mental stress of life in space. It can be taken for a longer time than Asian ginseng, since it is less stimulating. Regular consumption of the extract of this herb provides endurance and the capacity to handle heavy workloads with less strain on the body.

Besides protecting from stress, Siberian ginseng also increases oxygenation of the cells, thereby increasing endurance, alertness and visual-motor coordination. And it tones up the body while adjusting and normalising blood pressure and blood sugar levels. It has the rare ability to boost both immediate and long-term energy. Research shows Siberian ginseng to be effective in improving intellectual performance and enhancing mental stamina as well. This makes it useful in the elderly, particularly when combined with ginkgo.

When you're overworked, exhausted or involved in taxing tasks such as long-distance driving, performances, or coping with a hangover, ginseng is an ideal antidote. In these cases, short-term use is all you need to get you through the emergency. It can be used safely in the long term, as well, to help you cope with the stresses of daily life.

Siberian ginseng is taken at a dose of 200 to 400mg daily of standardised extract, containing greater than 1 per cent eleutherosides. The dose of tincture is 5ml twice daily of a 1:5 concentration (that is, five parts alcohol to one part ginseng).

Siberian ginseng is the safest and healthiest known stimulant, with generally no negative side-effects. It contains no steroid or other dangerous chemical agents. It does not have the depressing qualities or addictive potential of most other pharmacological and biological stimulants such as caffeine, amphetamines and cocaine. It doesn't 'stress' the system in stimulating it, and doesn't provoke any downregulation.

As with any substance, however, allergy can occur with ginseng. Menstrual abnormalities and breast tenderness have been reported by users of Asian ginseng, so for women, Siberian ginseng is often recommended instead. Over-use can cause over-stimulation, including insomnia in those who are in a more advanced stage of adrenal exhaustion. Unconfirmed reports of excessive doses raising blood pressure and increasing heart rate have been largely discredited. In traditional Chinese medicine ginseng is prescribed for pregnant women, but as with any herb this should be done only under the care of a health practitioner.

According to Chinese tradition, the best way to use ginseng is as part of a 2-month restoration programme. This is a time to gather and store energy, with a plan incorporating exercise, rest and relaxation, and avoidance of stress, drugs and alcohol. Coupled with regular ginseng intake, such a programme helps to build reserves of energy and vitality. Traditional sources recommend that you take a short break from ginseng after this renewal period. After that, it can be used as a tonic as needed. The German Commission E, a body similar to the US Food and Drug Administration (FDA), concurs, recommending no more than 3 months at a time on any of the ginsengs, including Siberian.

Maureen's case is a good example of the appropriate use of ginseng.

Maureen, a 40-year-old actress complained of being exhausted for the past 6 months. She had trouble sleeping, couldn't get out of bed in the morning, and would collapse after only 15 minutes of light exercise. Her doctor gave her Siberian ginseng (200mg, twice daily), along with licorice root and reishi mushrooms. Within 4 weeks, she was sleeping well and felt rested and able to get up easily in the morning. She was even able to exercise moderately for 30 minutes with no fatigue.

Siberian and Asian Ginseng

How they work: Adaptogenic, they support the adrenal glands.

Positive effects:
▶ Enhance the body's response to stress
▶ Decrease feelings of anxiety and stress
▶ Increase immediate energy (stimulant)
▶ Restore vitality, energy and endurance over time (tonic)
▶ Increase mental and physical performance.

Cautions: None for Siberian ginseng. For Asian ginseng, possible menstrual abnormalities and breast tenderness. Over-use may cause over-stimulation, including insomnia in sensitive individuals. Take a 1-month break after 3 months of taking ginseng.

How much?:
▶ Siberian ginseng, 200–400mg daily
▶ Asian ginseng, 100–200mg daily of a standardised extract containing 4 to 7 per cent ginsenosides.

Ashwaganda: Indian ginseng

A herb from India used in traditional Ayurvedic medicine, ashwaganda (*Withania somnifera*), also known as Indian ginseng, is increasingly being integrated into Western herbal practice. It is a versatile adaptogen. It can enhance the immune system, boost energy, calm the stress response and reduce levels of the stress hormone cortisol. It can also enhance memory and cognition due to its antioxidant effect and ability to increase acetylcholine receptor activity. On top of all this, it's an aphrodisiac!

It also increases thyroid hormone levels and basal body temperature – speeding up the metabolism – in some patients. In a study on animals with arthritis, ashwaganda proved better at reducing symptoms than hydrocortisone, suggesting that it has potent effects on adrenal hormone balance.

Ashwaganda

How it works: Adaptogen, stabilises cortisol levels, acetylcholine enhancer.

Positive effects: Energising, calming, reduces high cortisol levels, enhances libido, memory and cognition.

Cautions: None.

How much?: 300mg of a standardised extract, providing 1.5 per cent of withanolides, two to three times daily.

Licorice: balancing act

Licorice root (*Glycyrrhiza glabra*) provides support for the adrenal glands, helping with mild adrenal insufficiency and hypoglycaemia. It is also used in women for its oestrogen-balancing properties. It stimulates the adrenal cortex to elevate cortisol and adrenal sex hormones by preventing their breakdown. So if you take licorice, the cortisol you make lasts longer. While we have repeatedly talked about cortisol as negative, it is essential in the short-term handling of stress. Only under chronic stress does it become a problem.

Licorice helps to raise low blood pressure, which often accompanies chronic fatigue, but this can also lead to hypertension (high blood pressure) in susceptible individuals. To avoid this side-effect, the deglycyrrhinised form is used in many instances, such as in treating ulcers, but then the hormonal effect is lost.

Licorice

How it works: Prevents the breakdown of cortisol, thereby raising its level.

Positive effects: Improves adrenal function if exhausted, and raises low blood pressure.

Cautions: Can raise blood pressure in susceptible individuals. Not recommended for those with raised cortisol levels.

How much?: 500mg twice a day, morning and midday, not in the evening.

Reishi mushroom

The glossy red or black cap of this Chinese mushroom looks unusual, especially to Western eyes. Inside are phytochemicals that make it one of the most respected tonics in herbal medicine. In Asia, especially China and Japan, it has been revered for 5,000 years. Chinese reishi mushroom (*Ganodermum lucidum*) is often used to modify or enhance the effects of other stress-fighting herbs. With multiple benefits, it has no significant side-effects.

You can use it to calm your mind, sharpen your thinking and energise you when you are fatigued. It can even lower high blood pressure. Says herbalist Christopher Hobbs, 'I often take reishi myself and have experienced immediate calming and sleep-promoting effects. I have noticed an amazing feeling in my chest with some reishi extracts, as if my heart area has "opened up". This unique effect, while not scientifically proven, is entirely enjoyable and often is accompanied by a feeling of immediate serenity.' This certainly sounds like a natural high!

Reishi Mushroom

How it works: Acts as an adaptogen, stabilising adrenal hormones.

Positive effects: Both calming and energising, lowers blood pressure, sharpens mental function.

Cautions: None.

How much?: In tincture form (20 per cent) 10ml, three times a day; tablets 1000mg, 1–3 tablets three times a day.

Rhodiola

Another amazing adaptogen from the East with a long history of use is rhodiola. Growing in the Arctic regions of eastern Siberia, it is often called Arctic root. Folklore says that 'those who drank rhodiola tea regularly will live more than 100 years'. Chinese emperors, in search of the elixir of life, would send expeditions to Siberia to bring back this potent herb.

But it isn't all folklore. Modern science has confirmed that rhodiola has many proven benefits. Among these are its ability to improve energy, balance stress hormones, improve mood and boost your immunity. As an adaptogen it appears to be at least as powerful as ginseng, and protects against high levels of the stress hormone cortisol. However, it also stimulates both mental and physical performance. For this reason it was used in the Soviet Union to improve athletic powers.

Rhodiola's effects on the brain are perhaps the most interesting. Numerous studies have shown it to improve concentration, especially when tired. In one proof-reading test those taking rhodiola decreased their number of errors by 88 per cent! It also helps the brain make serotonin, which we shall learn is a key 'happy' neurotransmitter (see page 107). In one study 128 people suffering from depression were given 200mg of rhodiola. Two-thirds of the patients (65 per cent) had major reduction or disappearance of their symptoms. On top of this, rhodiola boosts immunity and has proven anti-cancer properties.

As with other herbs, make sure you are getting the real thing. There are many plant varieties of rhodiola, but the one that works is called *Rhodiola rosea*. While it has many active ingredients the key components are called rosavin and salidroside. So it is best to take rhodiola supplements that are standardised, and can therefore guarantee at least 2 per cent rosavin and 1 per cent salidroside.

Rhodiola (*Rhodiola rosea*)

How it works: Acts as an adaptogen stabilising adrenal hormones and promoting serotonin production.

Positive effects: Improves concentration, stress resistance, physical performance and mood. Boosts immunity.

Cautions: None.

How much?: 200–300mg daily of a standardised extract with meals

Stimulating amino acids: liven up your brain

Certain amino acids are essential for brain function because they provide the building blocks (precursors) for neurotransmitters and hormones. Essential, too, are the vitamin and mineral co-factors needed to convert the amino acids into neurotransmitters (see page 97). The key brain amino acids that stimulate are phenylalanine and tyrosine. They raise mood, energy, sexual interest, mental performance and memory.

Since amino acids are found in high-protein foods including meat, fish and eggs, you might think that the way to increase your amino acid levels would simply be to eat more of these foods. However, each protein supplies different combinations of amino acids. People who have specific amino acid deficiencies or increased needs due to prolonged stress, for instance, will require more specific supplementation.

For the best results, follow the instructions below for each of the amino acids. Since certain amino acids compete with others for transport into the brain, they are best taken separately.

Phenylalanine: natural caffeine

Found in meats, wheatgerm, dairy products, granola, chocolate and oat flakes, phenylalanine is an essential amino acid. It is converted by the body into tyrosine, which in turn is converted to the neurotransmitters dopamine, noradrenalin and adrenalin. It acts like natural caffeine, but without the downside.

Phenylalanine becomes depleted in cases of chronic stress and burnout, as well as by over-use of stimulant drugs such as cocaine, speed and nicotine. It helps alleviate symptoms of withdrawal, since it restores normal brain chemistry.

Supplements of this amino acid are available in three different forms: DL-phenylalanine (DLPA), D-phenylalanine and L-phenylalanine (see Supplement Directory, page 311). The D- and DL-forms have been proven to act as natural pain killers.[8] They enhance the action of endorphins and enkephalins, the natural opiates that reduce pain and produce feelings of well-being, even euphoria. Although some effect is felt within days, the full effect takes a few weeks to build up.

L-phenylalanine combines with vitamin B6 to produce phenethylamine, the stimulating 'love drug' that we find in chocolate (see page 79). One study from 1986 showed that 31 of 40 depressed patients with low levels of phenethylamine responded well to large doses of L-phenylalanine (up to 14g a day),[9] making it a very acceptable antidepressant – and, by extension, an antidote for chocolate cravings. In a double-blind study reported in 1979, DLPA (150–200mg a day) or the antidepressant imipramine was administered to 40 depressed patients (20 in each group) for 1 month. Both groups had the same positive result, with no statistical difference found between the two groups using both objective and subjective tests.[10]

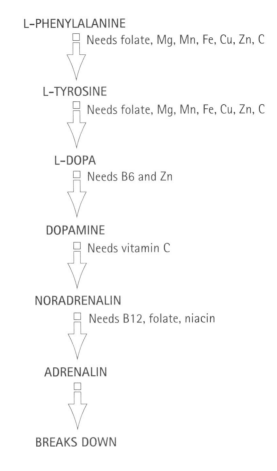

How dopamine, adrenalin and noradrenalin are made
from amino acids together with vitamins and minerals

Too much L-phenylalanine and to a lesser extent DLPA can cause overstimulation, anxiety, insomnia and hypertension (elevated blood pressure). When this happens, you should lower the dose, and if symptoms persist, stop it altogether. Overall, the best form to use is DLPA, since it is the most comprehensive and least expensive.

If you are low in DLPA or tyrosine you may feel tired and slow, and have trouble concentrating. You may also find it hard to get out of bed in the morning. A dose of either amino acid can help get you mobilised.

The effective dose is usually 500 to 1000mg of DLPA on an empty stomach first thing in the morning. However, everyone has different needs so it is better to start with about half the contents of a 500mg capsule, taken alone. For quick absorption, open the capsule and put the powder under your tongue. Watch your energy and mood go up. You will also need 25 to 50mg of vitamin B6 and 500mg of vitamin C to enhance its conversion to tyrosine.

DL-phenylalanine (DLPA)

How it works: Precursor for tyrosine, which converts to dopamine, adrenalin and noradrenalin.

Positive effects: Enhances mood, promotes energy, relieves pain and controls appetite.

Cautions: Can be too stimulating, causing anxiety, high blood pressure or insomnia. Should not be taken by people who have the metabolic disease phenylketonuria. Not recommended for those with a history of mania or mental illness.

How much?: 500–1000mg of DLPA on an empty stomach first thing in the morning. Can be repeated later in the day, but not too close to bedtime.

Tyrosine: big performer

Tyrosine is made in the body from phenylalanine, and has the same effects in the brain. It usually acts more rapidly, as it is one step further down the metabolic line. It readily crosses the blood-brain barrier to produce the energising neurotransmitters dopamine, noradrenalin and adrenalin. It is also used to make thyroid hormone, the body's energy controller, which manages both metabolic rate and energy production. When your thyroid function is low, so is your energy.

Some people find DLPA more effective than tyrosine for stimulation, but remember that in some people DLPA is more likely to cause hypertension (high blood pressure). DLPA also differs in controlling appetite by releasing CCK, an appetite suppressant made in the gut, and in acting as a pain reliever.

Neither amino acid should be taken with MAOIs (see page 113), a kind of antidepressant involving certain food restrictions, or by phenylketonurics, by those with malignant melanomas, or during pregnancy and breast-feeding.

Tyrosine has long been known by the military to improve mental and physical performance under stress. Research by the US military found that soldiers given tyrosine in stressful conditions of extreme cold, or while undertaking intense physical activity over prolonged periods of time, showed clear improvements in both mental and physical endurance. More recent research from Holland demonstrates how tyrosine gives you the edge in conditions of stress. A total of 21 cadets were put through a demanding 1-week military-combat-training course; 10 of them were given a drink containing 2g of tyrosine a day, while the remaining 11 were given an identical drink without the tyrosine. Those on tyrosine consistently performed better, both in memorising the task at hand and in tracking the tasks they had performed.[11]

Since individual sensitivity varies, start with 100mg or so of tyrosine (see Supplement Directory, page 311), even if it means partially emptying out a capsule, and work your way up to your ideal dose. You can take another dose later in the day when your energy is flagging, since DLPA and tyrosine are good, quick energisers. If you are feeling like you need a caffeine boost, open a 500mg DLPA or tyrosine capsule and put half of the contents under your tongue. It will be quickly absorbed, and give you the kick you want, without the rebound. You may need a whole one, but best to try half first. This avoids too much of a rush if you are particularly sensitive to its effects.

In response to regular usage, your brain actually produces more dopamine receptors to 'receive' this amino acid. This will raise mood over time in those with depression related to insufficient dopamine receptors, as in 'Reward Deficiency Syndrome' (see page 110). On the other hand, if you don't need it regularly, it's better to take it as needed for a good boost. In clinical practice, we measure the client's amino acid levels and determine if he or she actually needs to supplement. We then supplement, often in higher than the doses mentioned here, and monitor to be sure that balance is maintained.

Tyrosine

How it works: Precursor to stimulating neurotransmitters dopamine, adrenalin, noradrenalin and thyroid hormone, thyroxine.

Positive effects: Enhances mood, promotes energy and motivation, supports healthy thyroid function.

Cautions: Hypertension in those susceptible. Should not be taken by phenylketonurics, those with melanomas or pregnant or nursing women. Not recommended for those with a history of mania, unless under a doctor's care.

How much?: 500–1000mg on an empty stomach first thing in the morning, to prevent competition from other amino acids.

Other stimulants: best of the rest

NADH

NADH, or nicotinamide adenine dinucleotide, is a small organic molecule found naturally in every living cell. It is necessary for thousands of biochemical reactions within the body, playing a key role in the energy production of cells, particularly in the brain and central nervous system. It stimulates cellular production of the neurotransmitters dopamine, noradrenalin and serotonin, improving mental clarity, alertness and concentration. The more NADH a cell has available, the more energy it can produce, and the more efficiently it can perform. It also enhances physical performance and energy. We have found it very useful in the treatment of chronic fatigue syndrome.

NADH

How it works: Stimulates cellular production of the neurotransmitters dopamine, noradrenalin and serotonin.

Positive effects: Improves mental clarity, cellular memory, alertness and concentration. Is a good antioxidant, and enhances energy and athletic endurance.

Cautions: None.

How much?: 2.5–10mg daily, depending on individual requirements.

Green tea

Green tea contains certain important health-giving compounds. These polyphenols or catechins are potent antioxidants, with cancer-protective and anti-ageing effects. Tea also has a blood-thinning effect, similar to that of aspirin. As it turns out, black tea, a fermented form of the same leaf, also contains these compounds, but with proportionately more caffeine along with them. Green tea contains only 20 to 30mg of caffeine per cup, as compared to 50mg in a regular cup of tea, and is consequently less stimulating, even relaxing to many people. In fact, Asian monks have traditionally used it to help keep them awake, though still calm, during meditation practice.

Considering the health benefits, we can count green tea, in moderation (meaning two cups a day), as an acceptable 'natural stimulant'.

Green Tea

How it works: Contains potent antioxidants (see page 32).

Positive effects: Lowers cholesterol and blood pressure, increases HDL, the so-called 'good' cholesterol, thins the blood, reduces risk of heart attack, stroke and cancer, enhances immune function, prevents dental caries and hypertension, and aids weight loss by encouraging the body to burn fat.

Cautions: Green tea contains caffeine, so limit your intake.

How much?: Two cups a day.

Action Plan for Natural Stimulation

The first steps to maximising your natural energy and motivation are to reduce your stress level, balance your blood sugar, and avoid or reduce your intake of stimulants to an absolute minimum. A good all-round multi-vitamin supplement is key. You'll need to follow the advice in Chapter 3, 'Natural High Basics' and Chapter 4, 'Relaxants'. Part Three, 'Living High Naturally', also gives you plenty of energy-generating exercises.

The key to naturally stimulating supplements are the adaptogens. Asian ginseng can, however, be over-stimulating if you have very raised cortisol levels or are exhausted. The same caution does not apply to Siberian ginseng. Licorice can also be over-stimulating so don't supplement it if you are very stressed or exhausted.

The following nutrients are worthy additions to a supplement programme designed to enhance your energy and motivation. The combination, taken every day, is likely to improve your mental and physical energy, stamina and motivation.

NATURAL STIMULANT	COMBINED	ALONE
Siberian ginseng*	100mg	200mg
Asian/American ginseng*	100mg	200mg
Ashwaganda*	400mg	900mg
Rhodiola*	100mg	200mg
Reishi mushroom	300mg	1000mg
DLPA	150mg	500mg
Tyrosine	150mg	500mg
Pantothenic acid	100mg	250mg

*Please note: all amounts given for herbs are for specified standardised extracts.

Take the following to feel alert and energetic

▶ A good all-round multivitamin supplying optimal amounts of B vitamins, especially pantothenic acid (vitamin B5), and vitamin C (see Chapter 3, 'Natural High Basics').

▶ A 'stimulant' formula providing Siberian, American and Asian ginseng, ashwaganda, reishi mushroom, DLPA, tyrosine and pantothenic acid.

▶ Optional licorice as needed, but only if you are not seriously stressed, when you will have raised cortisol levels, and certainly not at night.

For a full natural energy-boost programme, see 'Top Tips' in Part Four.

◀6▶

MOOD ENHANCERS

UPBEAT, CHEERFUL and at peace with the world – it's a fantastic feeling, and we can't get enough of it. Sometimes literally: we're all prone to moods, and it's only natural to feel blue from time to time. Occasional bouts of sadness may even help us appreciate the good times! In any case, most of us will bounce back within a short time – hours, days, or even a week or two. For example, when Peter suddenly lost his job of 4 years, he felt disheartened for a couple of weeks. Then he found a new, and even better, job, and life was good again. In a similar vein, Lacey was distraught after breaking up with her boyfriend after 3 years together, but with the support of friends got over her feelings in a month.

It wasn't quite so simple, though, when Lacey's friend Janet broke up with *her* boyfriend. Janet was in tears for days on end, withdrew from friends and family, and felt like a total failure. Not only did her response seem out of proportion to the event, but she was on a downward spiral, heading towards clinical depression. In fact, Janet always had been more on the 'down' side, lacking the joie de vivre of her friend Lacey.

We all fit somewhere in this range, with most of us probably more or less able to take adversity in our stride. But what is it that makes some people less resilient than others? And are there ways to increase our ability to handle the slings and arrows that life flings at us?

We can assure you there are. In this chapter, we'll take a look at what happens to your brain chemistry when you're feeling blue. Then we'll cover the antidepressants commonly prescribed to counter these feelings. Finally, we will show you how to vanquish the blues safely, by using a number of natural mood enhancers that can elevate your spirits without the side-effects of drugs.

Mood Check

First, check yourself out on the questionnaire below, to find out where you fit on the continuum, from happy and content, to blue, all the way down to clinically depressed. (No one but you will be looking at the answers, so be honest!)

Score 1 for each 'yes' answer.

HOW BLUE ARE YOU?	YES	NO
Do you feel downhearted, blue and sad?	☐	☐
Do you feel worse in the morning?	☐	☐
Do you have crying spells, or feel like it?	☐	☐
Do you have trouble falling asleep, or sleeping through the night?	☐	☐
Is your appetite poor?	☐	☐
Are you losing weight without trying?	☐	☐
Do you feel unattractive and unlovable?	☐	☐
Do you prefer to be alone?	☐	☐
Do you feel fearful?	☐	☐
Are you often tired and irritable?	☐	☐
Is it an effort to do the things you used to do?	☐	☐
Are you restless and unable to keep still?	☐	☐
Do you feel hopeless about the future?	☐	☐
Do you find it difficult to make decisions?	☐	☐
Do you feel less enjoyment from activities that once gave you pleasure?	☐	☐

If your score is:

Below 5: You are normal. You appear to be positive, optimistic and able to roll with the punches. This chapter will give you clues on how to handle those occasions when things aren't going so well for you.

5 to 10: You have a mild to moderate case of the blues. Read on to see how this can happen, and then, to the solutions. You might also consider seeking outside help.

More than 10: You are moderately to markedly depressed. Beside reading this chapter, you should seek outside help.

If you were in the depressed range, you should start by consulting your physician or health practitioner to make sure there is no physical cause for your problems. Once you've done that, consult both a psychotherapist and a natural medicine practitioner (see Resources, page 304). One will deal with psychological issues, while the other will help to find any underlying chemical imbalance that might be causing the problem.

Feed your brain, beat the blues

In any case, if you are depressed, don't feel stigmatised. Depression affects more than three million people in Britain and is on the increase worldwide. Moreover, the condition is often biochemical, which is why current treatment approaches include drug therapy as well as psychotherapy.

What is most often overlooked, however, is that mood, behaviour and mental performance all depend on a variety of nutrients that both make up and fuel the brain, nervous system and neurotransmitters. So a low mood may have less to do with past trauma or a faulty belief system than with deficient nutrients. We've already encountered a number of these, which include vitamins B3, B6, folic acid (folate), B12 and C, zinc, magnesium, essential fatty acids, and the amino acids, tryptophan and tyrosine.

Research at King's College Hospital, London, for example, found that 33 per cent of those with psychiatric disorders, including depression, were deficient in the B vitamin folate.[1] Other surveys of depressed patients found that many were deficient in iron or B vitamins, especially folate. It seems a shame that, with such a simple solution, so many people are suffering needlessly. What is more worrisome is that government dietary surveys show that a large portion of the population doesn't get even the bare minimum, the recommended daily amount (RDA) of these vitamins and minerals, in their daily diet. It is no wonder that depression is on the increase!

So, if we're poorly nourished, we're actually less able to cope with life's challenges. Once we're eating the way we should, our mood goes up, and we can handle life's events more resiliently. A good analogy can be found in Dr Ray Sahelian's book, *Mind Boosters*. He compares a happy, healthy mind to a pond with a high water level, representing brain chemicals. There may be many rocks of all shapes and sizes below the tranquil surface. These represent the hurts and traumas that are a part of life. If the water becomes depleted, these rocks begin to show, and the previously submerged pain comes to the surface. We need to keep those brain chemicals topped up.

That's not the whole story, however. Taking too much of the wrong substances is just as damaging as failing to take the right ones, and sugar and stimulants top the list of no-nos. You'll recall how blood sugar imbalances, often related to excessive sugar, alcohol or caffeine intake, can stimulate neurotransmitter release and a quick high. Not for long, though: the brain responds to an ongoing use of sugar, as with any drug, by downregulating, leaving you with insufficient feel-good chemicals. There's no doubt that stress, over-use of stimulants and blood sugar problems are a major contributor to low moods. Certain medications, including antihistamines, tranquillisers, sleeping pills, narcotics and recreational drugs, can also interfere with your neurotransmitters, leading to depression.

How then, do we take on the care and feeding of our brains? We need to start with the key neurotransmitters serotonin and noradrenalin – if these aren't in balance, they can cause depression and low moods. Both antidepressant drugs and supplements aim to enhance their actions. In fact, a great deal of our information comes from the extensive pharmaceutical research done in the past few decades to develop new antidepressant medications.

Serotonin and noradrenalin have different roles in countering depression. Depression can be felt as extreme unhappiness or as a lack of drive or motivation, and people can feel more of one or the other, or a mixture of both. Using a psychological test called the Social Adaptation Self-evaluation Scale, a 1998 study found that a serotonin-enhancing drug had most effect on self-image and mood, while noradrenalin was more involved in promoting motivation and drive.[2] We will soon see that there are ways to attain these results without taking drugs.

Serotonin: the mood neurotransmitter

Serotonin is considered the 'mood neurotransmitter' which keeps us emotionally and socially stable. It is interesting to note that women seem to have more problems than men in maintaining their serotonin levels. Yes, women are moodier – and this is not a sexist comment, but just a reflection of biological truth, likely due to the interplay between serotonin and the female hormone cycle. This would explain the emotional shifts related to menstrual periods, when many women experience increased moodiness, irritability and sensitivity to pain. Women who are low in serotonin are likelier to express their anger inwardly, with depression and even suicidal behaviour.

Research shows that, in contrast, men who are low in serotonin are often violent and can even engage in dangerous criminal acts. Alcohol and drug abusers also turn out to be low in serotonin. The good news is that we can successfully correct these imbalances by supplying supplements that raise serotonin.

'Good mood' foods: the tryptophan connection

Serotonin comes from the essential amino acid tryptophan, which is found in protein-containing foods such as fish, turkey, chicken, cottage cheese, avocados, bananas and wheatgerm. Researchers have found that when they take recovered depressed patients and deprive them of tryptophan, their depression returns. As we saw in Chapter 2 (page 14), this has been well demonstrated by research at Oxford University's Department of Psychiatry. Women with a history of depression were divided into two groups, and given a diet excluding or including tryptophan under double-blind conditions (that is, neither the subjects nor the researchers knew who received which diet). At the end of the experiment, 10 out of 15 women on the tryptophan-free diet were significantly depressed, while no one on the tryptophan diet had any problem at all.[3] When the deprived group was given diets containing tryptophan, their depression lifted.

In general, giving tryptophan to depressed people has been beneficial, although some trials have not found it had a significant effect when compared with a placebo.[4] One possible explanation is that, without sufficient B3 and B6, tryptophan can be processed along a different chemical pathway, turning into a substance called kynurenine instead of serotonin (see opposite).

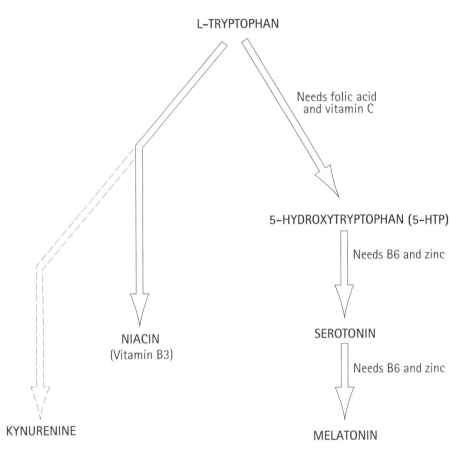

How the essential amino acid tryptophan can transform into the good-mood chemical serotonin, as well as melatonin

For this reason, supplementing an amino acid called 5-hydroxytryptophan, which is one step closer to turning into serotonin, has been shown to produce even better mood-enhancing results. These remarkable results are explained in more detail on page 120.

Noradrenalin: be rewarded

The neurotransmitter noradrenalin gives us feelings of motivation and of pleasure. While, like the stress hormone adrenalin, it is derived from dopamine, noradrenalin is more involved with positive stress states such as being in love, the thrill of music and dancing and other exhilarating and stimulating pursuits. As we mentioned in Chapter 5, some people inherit a gene that makes them deficient in these neurotransmitters, leaving them more prone to depression. They also crave stimulation from sugar, coffee, stress and alcohol. Described by researcher Kenneth Blum as 'Reward Deficiency Syndrome', its victims have a hard time feeling good, or 'rewarded', under normal conditions. Blum discovered that they can ingest the precursor amino acids tyrosine and phenylalanine, which, with the help of vitamin co-factors, convert to dopamine. This enhances mood and motivation and even reduces craving for the addictive substances. You don't have to have RDS to benefit from them, however. Many people are deficient for various reasons, and feel better once levels are normalised.

So much for how your brain stays happy. Now we'll take a look at the antidepressants on offer that claim to chase the blues away.

Antidepressants: The Pros and Cons

Researchers began developing a number of synthetic drugs for the treatment of depression in the 1950s – and they took off in a big way. At the time, they were seen as a breakthrough. Many different antidepressant medications are now available. They fall into four principal classes, distinguished by how they differ in affecting the balance and function of specific neurotransmitters: the tricyclic drugs, the monoamine oxidase inhibitors (MAOIs), the selective serotonin re-uptake inhibitors (SSRIs) and the noradrenalin re-uptake inhibitor drugs (NARIs). There are also three other antidepressant drugs that are chemically distinct both from these types and from each other: buproprion (Wellbutrin), trazodone (Desyrel) and venlaxafine (Effexor).

Antidepressants have helped many desperate people live happier lives. However, these powerful medications have also been greatly overprescribed. In Hyla's book, *St John's Wort: Nature's Blues Buster*, she explains their use in great detail, and compares them to the natural products. You'll find a briefer treatment here. There is plenty of good scientific evidence that natural products will often work just as well, and without the side-effects.

The various types of antidepressants differ in their mechanisms of action and side-effects. The figure on page 112 explains how they work. However, they all have several things in common. They are effective in reducing depressive symptoms in 50 to 80 per cent of those who use them. They may take from 4 to 6 weeks to produce their full effects, although side-effects and changes in mood can occur much sooner. Tricyclics were the first antidepressant medications, dominating the market for some 20 years. Used less frequently now, they work in various ways to affect the actions of noradrenalin and serotonin. The box below reveals a number of frightening downsides to these drugs.

Downside of Tricyclics

▶ Can induce drowsiness, dizziness, heart palpitations, dry mouth, blurred vision, confusion, weight gain, sweating, rashes, nausea, constipation or diarrhoea, difficulty with urination, impotence or impaired erection in men, inhibited orgasm in women, nightmares and anxiety.

SSRIs: Prozac works, but the side-effects are depressing

Serotonin, 'the civilising neurotransmitter', plays a vital role in mood, memory, appetite, sleep, pain perception and sexual desire. Selective serotonin re-uptake inhibitors, or SSRIs, block the neuron's re-absorption of serotonin (see Chapter 2). This makes more of the neurotransmitter available, with a resulting elevation in mood. Currently prescribed SSRIs include fluoxetine (Prozac), fluvoxamine (Luvox, Faverin), paroxetine (Paxil, Seroxat), sertraline (Zoloft, Lustral) and citalopram (Cipramil, Celexa).

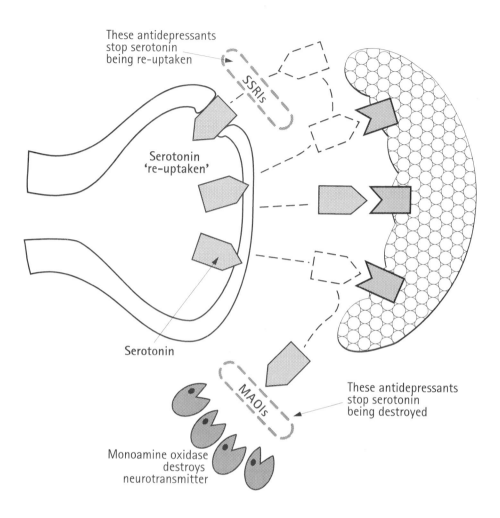

These antidepressants
stop serotonin
being re-uptaken

SSRIs

Serotonin
're-uptaken'

Serotonin

These antidepressants
stop serotonin
being destroyed

MAOIs

Monoamine oxidase
destroys
neurotransmitter

How antidepressants keep neurotransmitters delivering messages

While the SSRIs don't have the same side-effects as the tricyclics, they do bring their own problems. First, they often compromise libido and sexual performance in most people, men and women alike. Second, they are not euphoriants, but rather mood-stabilisers, even mood-flatteners. They often limit the highs along with the lows, and many people taking them end up with a zombie-like lack of emotion, as well as a host of other side-effects (see box opposite).

Here is what one Prozac user's husband had to say.

My wife was on Prozac. It led her to have an 'I don't give a darn' attitude about important things, and she had stomach pain the entire time she was on it. She then went off Prozac and started on St John's wort. The stomach problems went away the day she stopped Prozac. Now that she's on St John's wort, her depression hasn't returned. She is relaxed with a caring attitude.

And here is what Jan, herself prescribed SSRIs, had to say.

I've suffered from 'the blues' all my life. I took the antidepressant Zoloft, 100mg twice a day. It worked, but it was expensive and I couldn't stand the side-effects. I am also not sure I liked the levelling off of all my emotions! So, a month ago I began substituting St John's wort, two tablets at night instead of the Zoloft. I'm very happy with the results. I no longer suffer debilitating PMS, either.

Downside of Prozac and Other SSRIs

▶ Compromise libido and sexual performance in men and women.

▶ Can 'flatten' moods to the point of zombie-like emotionlessness.

▶ Can bring on forty-five other side-effects, including nausea, nervousness, insomnia, headache, tremors, anxiety, drowsiness, dry mouth, excessive sweating and diarrhoea.

The monoamine oxidase inhibitors: watch the pressure

The monoamine oxidase inhibitors, or MAOIs, work by reducing the quantity within the synapses of the enzyme MAO (monoamine-oxidase).

Since it ordinarily breaks down neurotransmitters, its reduction leads to higher adrenalin and dopamine levels. The most common are phenelzine sulfate (Nardil) and tranylcypromine sulfate (Parnate). They can produce a dangerous elevation in blood pressure if the patient takes decongestants, antihistamine or foods containing the amino acid tyramine. This is called the 'cheese effect' because that is one of the common foods that can cause this interaction.

Downside of MAOIs

▶ If MAOIs are taken with decongestants, antihistamine or foods containing tyramine, such as cheese or red wine, dangerously high blood pressure can result.

Other antidepressants

There are some antidepressants that don't fit the above categories: bupropion (Wellbutrin), trazodone (Desyrel), and venlafaxine (Effexor), but also appear to affect neurotransmitter activity.

All this said, there is a role for medications as well as herbs in psychiatric treatment. There are circumstances when one or the other is called for, and there are situations when they are needed in combination. However, the synthetic pharmaceutical medications should be reserved for those times when their benefits outweigh their costs. During Hyla's years of clinical practice, she learned that natural supplements should be the first line of treatment. Their more gentle actions are often all that is needed to resolve the imbalances leading to depression, as you will see next.

Natural Blues-busters

Many people prone to depression have found that they can control their moods very well with natural supplements which lack the side-effects of antidepressant drugs. You have to know what to take, and what effects to expect, however.

While SSRIs and the like tend to increase the supply of neurotransmitter by inhibiting re-uptake, or by preventing their breakdown, nutritional supplements provide raw 'construction' materials. If your mood problems are due to a deficiency in the materials that make up the neurotransmitters, then simply inhibiting their re-uptake won't solve your problem in the long run. That is why the drugs often stop working after a while.

The key mood-enhancing herbs and nutrients are:

▶ St John's wort
▶ Tryptophan and 5-HTP
▶ Phenylalanine and tyrosine (see Chapter 5)
▶ SAMe and TMG
▶ Omega-3 fats – EPA and DHA
▶ B vitamins, vitamin C and zinc.

We have provided a diagram overleaf that shows how our brain makes and maintains the right balance of neurotransmitters that enhance our mood and keep us motivated. Ensuring an optimal intake of these nutrients is the best way to stay happy.

St John's wort: wonder weed

An antidepressant that's as effective as the drugs, but has mild side-effects, if any, and even boosts libido? Sounds like fantasy? No: you've just met St John's wort, a herb taken by many thousands of people in Europe alone. In fact, *Hypericum perforatum* is prescribed by European doctors five times as often as Prozac.

Animal studies show that St John's wort inhibits the re-uptake of serotonin, and possibly also dopamine and noradrenalin. It appears to act like both the SSRIs and tricyclic antidepressants, but without their side-effects.

A 1996 review of 23 randomised clinical trials on St John's wort, involving 1,700 people in total, showed an equivalent response to

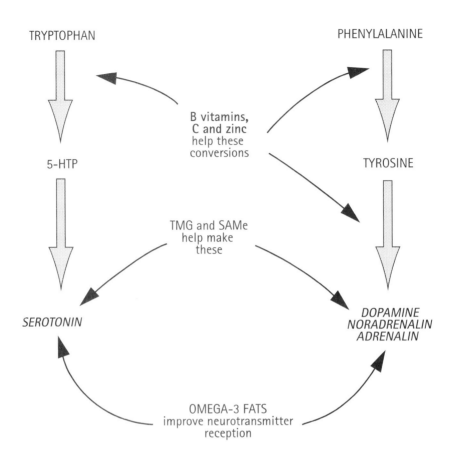

How mood–enhancing nutrients keep you motivated and happy

antidepressants with minimal side-effects.[5] At a dose of 300mg a day of a 0.3 per cent hypericin extract, St John's wort appears to help those with mild to moderate depression. There is even some evidence that doubling this dose can help those with severe depression.[6] St John's wort is also useful in calming your nerves, and in helping you to sleep more soundly.

While hypericin has been generally accepted as the likely active ingredient, there is evidence that the active antidepressant ingredient may actually be hyperforin. As a result, you may begin to see more St John's wort products on the market that are standardised to hyperforin (as well as to the usual hypericin).

St John's Wort vs Antidepressant Drugs

▶ Its side-effects are not nearly as severe or frequent.

▶ Mixing with alcohol doesn't lead to adverse reactions, as with the other antidepressants.

▶ It is not addictive.

▶ It does not produce withdrawal symptoms when you stop.

▶ It does not produce habituation, or the need for increased dosages to maintain its effects.

▶ It can be easily stopped and restarted without requiring a long build-up period.

▶ It enhances sleep and dreaming.

▶ It does not inhibit sex drive as SSRIs do in some people – and can actually enhance it in others.

▶ It does not make you sleepy in the daytime. In fact, it has shown in experiments to enhance alertness and driving reaction time.

▶ According to one report, the annual rate of death by overdose on antidepressant drugs is 30.1 per 1 million prescriptions. No one has ever died from an overdose of St John's wort. In fact, we don't think anyone has even tried to OD with it!

Because St John's wort was originally believed to work through MAO inhibition (see page 113), some articles still list the MAOI food restrictions. However, it is now quite clear that St John's wort in normal doses does not have this effect. But there are a number of cautions associated with the herb, as you'll see from the box below. To put it into perspective, though: many common drugs *and even grapefruit juice* will have a similar effect, since they activate the same liver enzymes as St John's wort.

St John's Wort

How it works: It appears to inhibit re-uptake of the neurotransmitters serotonin, noradrenalin and dopamine, and enhances GABA activity as well.

Positive effects: Enhances mood, acts as an antidepressant, combats anxiety in most, and helps you to sleep.

Cautions: May cause allergic reactions, rashes, gastrointestinal problems, sun sensitivity in susceptible individuals. Can cause anxiety or insomnia in certain people if taken too close to bedtime. Can reduce the potency of protease inhibitors (taken as treatment for AIDS) or cyclosporin (an immunosuppressant taken by organ transplant patients), digoxin (heart medication), or even, possibly, birth control pills. There is no proof as yet for this last one. St John's wort has not been researched sufficiently to recommend it for use in pregnancy and nursing. If combined with 5-HTP (see below), there's the possibility of serotonin syndrome – headache, an increase in body temperature and heavy sweating. Seek medical advice if this occurs.

How much?: 300mg of an extract of 0.3 per cent hypericin, starting with one or two capsules/tablets in the morning with breakfast. If there is no change after a week, add a third dose at lunch. You can also take it as doses of 450mg each, or take your entire daily dose in the morning, since the effect lasts for a long time.

Tryptophan: back from the brink

We've already read a bit on tryptophan. But what about taking it as a supplement? A once popular over-the-counter treatment for depression and insomnia, L-tryptophan was banned in the US by the Food and Drug Administration in 1989, and shortly thereafter in Britain, after a contaminated batch from Japan caused a serious illness called eosinophilia myalgia syndrome. Despite the fact that the exact cause of this outbreak was determined to be due to specific contamination, the FDA persisted in their declaration that L-tryptophan itself was unsafe. In this context it's curious that it continued to be available in infant formulas and intravenous feedings. One can at least speculate that the explanation for such an obvious inconsistency can be found in the enormous financial and political influence of pharmaceuticals companies.

L-tryptophan, which is currently only available on prescription, usually comes in 500mg capsules, and the recommended dose is 1000mg, or up to 2000mg daily. You can take 50mg or so in the morning, and 50 to 2000mg an hour before bedtime if you need help in falling asleep. The enzyme tryptophan hydroxylase, which converts tryptophan into 5-HTP, depends on folic acid and vitamin C. 5-HTP is turned into serotonin, with the aid of co-factors biotin, B6 and zinc, and the enzyme 5-HTP carboxylase. Make sure you are taking enough of these by supplementing a high potency multivitamin. Also, a carbohydrate snack such as fruit acts as a vehicle to transport it into the brain. Since other amino acids or proteins will compete for the same space, don't take tryptophan with protein-rich foods.

L-tryptophan

How it works: Raw material or precursor, for the neurotransmitter serotonin.

Positive effects: Promotes relaxation, elevated mood and deep sleep.

Cautions: May cause nausea, headaches, constipation and other gastrointestinal problems in certain people or with high doses. It should not be taken during pregnancy, with MAO inhibitors, or in cases of the autoimmune disease, lupus.

How much?: 500–2000mg daily, with 1000mg at bedtime, plus B vitamins and a little carbohydrate.

5-HTP (5-hydroxytryptophan): out of Africa

In 1995 5-HTP – the metabolite of tryptophan, a step further along in the metabolic pathway – became available as an extract from seeds of the African shrub griffonia. Like L-tryptophan, it converts to serotonin, inducing relaxation, elevated mood and sleep. It may be even more useful than tryptophan because much of the tryptophan we eat is processed along different biochemical pathways. 5-HTP, on the other hand, is a direct precursor of serotonin and enters the brain easily. Unlike tryptophan, it can be taken with food and other supplements, including amino acids, with no interference.

Not surprisingly, results treating depression with 5-HTP have proven more effective than tryptophan. For example, a double-blind trial headed by Dr Poldinger at the Basle University of Psychiatry gave 34 depressed patients 300mg of 5-HTP and 29 patients fluvoxamine (Prozac) which is a state-of-the-art SSRI antidepressant. Each patient was assessed for their degree of depression using the widely accepted Hamilton Rating Scale, plus their own subjective self-assessment. At the end of the 6 weeks, both groups of patient had had a significant improvement in their depression; however, those taking 5-HTP had had a greater improvement in each of the four criteria assessed – depression, anxiety, insomnia and physical symptoms, as well as the patient's self-assessment.[7] 5-HTP had outperformed the best antidepressant. Given that 5-HTP is less expensive and has significantly less side-effects, it is extraordinary that it is virtually never prescribed by psychiatrists.

5-HTP is about ten times more powerful than L-tryptophan, so the dose needed is one-tenth the L-tryptophan dose. It is available in 50 and 100mg capsules. For anxiety or depression, the dose is 50 to 200mg a day, taken in divided doses. You can take 50 to 200mg of this at bedtime if you're having trouble sleeping.

Some people report drowsiness if they take 5-HTP during the day, so use caution to determine your best daytime dose. Since there are few studies on the long-term effects, it is best taken for a month or two at a time only, with a few weeks off before restarting.

5-HTP

How it works: Precursor for the neurotransmitter serotonin.

Positive effects: Induces relaxation, elevated mood and sleep, and suppresses appetite.

Cautions: Nausea and gastrointestinal problems in high doses.

How much?: For daytime use: 50–100mg twice daily. For sleep: 50–100mg of the daily total dose at bedtime.

Phenylalanine and tyrosine: dynamic duo

These natural mood-boosters have already been covered extensively in Chapter 5. For a complete rundown on them and essential information on possible downsides, doses and so on, see pages 96 to 100. Phenylalanine and tyrosine are amino acid precursors to noradrenalin, adrenalin and dopamine.

Phenylalanine is converted to tyrosine, which is then converted to dopamine and then noradrenalin. They require as co-factor nutrients the vitamins niacin, B6, B12, folic acid and C, plus the minerals zinc, magnesium, copper, iron and manganese. The most effective form of phenylalanine for mood enhancement is DLPA, which has proven as effective as tricyclic antidepressants.

Most of the research on people's moods is done by pharmaceuticals companies while they are developing new drugs. First, laboratory animals are used in the experiments. Then people suffering from depression are recruited as their test subjects. As a result, we don't have much information on the effects of these substances in 'normal' people, who want to take products simply to boost their mood.

SAMe: turning on the lights

Recently, there has been a great deal of media attention about the natural compound SAMe (s-adenosyl-methionine), pronounced 'Sammy'. A new 'convert' to SAMe, 35-year-old Marisa, shared the following experience:

> I had been feeling just 'blah' for what seemed like years. I read about St John's wort and took it for a month, 300mg, three times daily. I felt somewhat better, but something was still missing. Then I added SAMe, 400mg a day. It's like someone turned on the lights. I felt like a kid again, playing, being happy, and not burdened as I had become.

For those of you with no mood problems, but just wanting to feel a little high, you can expect a similar experience. An appropriate dose (see below) on an empty stomach can put a spring in your step, a sparkle in your eye and a grin on your face.

Placebo-controlled, double-blind studies show that SAMe is equal or superior to antidepressants, and works faster, most often within a few days (most pharmaceutical antidepressants may take 3 to 6 weeks to take effect), and with no significant side-effects. Instead, SAMe has side benefits, including being an effective treatment for degenerative joint disease, fibromyalgia and liver problems. According to one comprehensive review of all the studies, 92 per cent of depressive patients responded to SAMe, compared with 85 per cent for the medications.[8]

If you stop taking SAMe suddenly, you'll experience no withdrawal reaction – a common pitfall when antidepressants are stopped abruptly. SAMe also protects your liver, in contrast to the potential liver damage triggered by older tricyclic antidepressants.

Except for the adrenal and pineal glands, the liver contains the most SAMe of any body organ. In the body the liver depends on SAMe for regeneration, detoxification, bile production, and the essential biochemical processes of both methylation and the production of glutathione, the liver's natural antioxidant. SAMe aids the liver in neutralising toxins, carcinogens and free radicals. This process slows the ageing process, including brain ageing.

That's not all. Research shows that SAMe treats the fatigue, inflammation and pain associated with fibromyalgia, a puzzling and hard-to-treat condition. Patients have reported significant benefits from taking 400 to 800mg of SAMe daily, including improved sleep, reduced fatigue, reduction in pain and enhanced mood. All-in-all, quite a remarkable nutrient!

How much should you take? Start with 200mg twice daily, taken on an empty stomach preferably an hour away before or after eating. If you experience nausea or gastrointestinal problems, reduce the dose and take it with meals, although the food will cut its potency somewhat. It's usually enough to take 400mg per day.

If you don't see results in a few days, you can gradually increase the dose, by 200mg every few days, up to a maximum of 400mg four times daily. Then, once your mood feels stable, you can reduce it gradually to a lower maintenance dose. In general, the longer SAMe is used, the more beneficial the results.

SAMe should be taken with its co-factors vitamins B6 (50mg), B12 (1000mcg) and folic acid (800mcg) to enhance production of the SAMe precursor, methionine. These vitamins can be taken separately, as part of your multivitamin regime.

Although the price is now coming down, SAMe has been quite expensive, with one 200mg tablet costing approximately £1. This could easily add up. Unfortunately, its cost has been a limiting factor in its distribution and overall use.

A word of caution. Though this effect is not reported in the literature, higher doses cause irritability, anxiety or insomnia in some people. In this case, lower the dose, but if the effect continues, stop taking it. By the same token, SAMe's antidepressant activity may trigger a manic phase in individuals with bipolar disorder, so they should not take SAMe unless under medical supervision. The same cautions apply to the use of TMG (below).

Trimethylglycine (TMG): more of the SAMe

An alternative to SAMe is trimethylglycine (TMG), also a methyl donor. The body can make SAMe directly from TMG, which is both stable and much less expensive. While it has not been as extensively researched as SAMe, the fact that it is a direct precursor of SAMe would predict that its effect would be very similar.

TMG is also known as glycine betaine, not to be confused with 'betaine hydrochloride', which is used to help increase stomach acid. A precursor to SAMe, TMG turns into homocysteine (a substance that in excess can be toxic to the heart), SAMe and methionine. This process also yields DMG (dimethylglycine), a well-known performance enhancer, which thus doubles TMG's benefits.

Extracted from sugar beet, TMG is also found in broccoli and spinach. Except for the cautions listed above, it has no reported side-effects other than brief muscle-tension headaches, and only if it is taken in large quantities without food. Optimal doses needed to raise SAMe are 1000 to 3000mg per day. In combined formulas, a 100 to 250mg dose is enough.

An important point is that SAMe and TMG, unlike many other natural and synthetic antidepressants, are safe to take during pregnancy and breast-feeding. There are also no reported negative interactions with other medications, such as antidepressants. This makes them particularly useful in the elderly who are often on a variety of medications, and are also more sensitive to side-effects. SAMe can be used safely with other natural supplements, too, including St John's wort.

SAMe (s-adenosyl-methionine)

How it works: Naturally occurring molecule, essential in the manufacture of neurotransmitters.

Positive effects: Enhances neurotransmitter activity, acts as a natural mood enhancer and stimulant.

Cautions: Higher doses may lead to irritability, anxiety, insomnia and nausea. SAMe's antidepressant activity may lead to the manic phase in individuals with bipolar disorder (manic depression), so they should be monitored carefully.

How much?: 200mg twice daily, on an empty stomach, increasing gradually to a maximum of 1000mg a day if needed.

Omega-3 brain fats: up with fish

On page 29 we saw how important the omega-3 fatty acids are for health. And, as it turns out, happiness. The omega-3 fatty acids, EPA and DHA, are found in oily, carnivorous fish such as herring, mackerel, tuna and salmon. It's notable that in countries where there is higher fish consumption, there is a lower rate of depression. Also, diets and drugs that severely lower cholesterol tend to exacerbate omega-3 deficiency, causing depression, whereas supplementing omega-3 fish oils has proven effective in elevating mood. There is also a correlation between the incidence of depression and heart disease, and both are associated with omega-3 fat deficiency. (For a fuller discussion of the research on the omega-3 fats see the discussion on natural mind and memory boosters on page 143.)

To ensure an optimal intake of the essential omega 3 brain fats, eat oily fish three times a week. Otherwise, take an omega-3 fish oil supplement providing 500 to 1000mg of EPA plus DHA daily. Most fish oil supplements provide around 400mg of EPA plus DHA so you'll need two a day. If you are vegan or vegetarian, eat a tablespoon of flaxseeds a day and one dessertspoon of flaxseed oil.

EPA and DHA

How they work: Building material for neuron membranes and neurotransmitter receptor sites, enhancing neural transmission and increasing serotonin levels.

Positive effects: Improve learning, memory and mood in depression, bipolar disorder and dyslexia.

Cautions: None.

How much?: 500–1000mg a day as a fish oil supplement, or eat oily fish three times a week.

B vitamins and minerals: food for thought

Some of your brain's best friends, the B vitamins have many roles to play in ensuring optimal brain function. They are vital for delivering oxygen to the brain and protecting it from harmful oxidants. They also help turn glucose into energy within brain cells, and help to keep neurotransmitters in circulation. Vitamins B6, B12 and folic acid are most important in terms of enhancing mood.

B6 (pyridoxine)

This has an important role in brain function – it's essential for the manufacture of neurotransmitters. It is also necessary for the conversion of amino acids into serotonin. A deficiency in this important neurotransmitter can cause depression and other problems. One study showed that about a fifth of depressed people who took part were deficient in pyridoxine.[9] We suggest you take 20 to 100mg a day.

B12 (cyanocobalamin)

B12 is very important for the health of nerve cells, and B12 deficiency is a major cause of mental deterioration and confusion in older people. You need 10 to 100mcg a day. Some people have very poor absorption of B12 and may benefit from much higher amounts, such as 1000mcg daily. B12 is easier to absorb in a formula designed to be taken under the tongue.

Folic acid (folate)

Like B12, this is essential for oxygen delivery to the brain. Deficiency in either results in anaemia. In high doses folic acid has been shown to substantially lessen depression and symptoms of schizophrenia.[10] You need about 400mcg daily.

It is important to remember that B vitamins should be taken in combination, or you could experience side-effects. For example, too much B6 on its own can cause neurological problems. So if you wish to supplement a specific B vitamin take this with a multivitamin containing all the B vitamins.

Action Plan for a Natural Mood Lift

From a biochemical perspective, here's what to do to enhance your mood, but do bear in mind that low moods can be due to psychological factors. These are discussed in Chapter 15, 'Positive Thinking'.

▶ Start with the Natural High Basics diet and supplements, including fish or flaxseed oil or a regular dietary intake of fish and/or flaxseeds. Your basic supplement programme needs to include a high-strength multivitamin and vitamin C, supplying optimal amounts of B vitamins (see 'Natural High Basics', page 33).

▶ Balance your blood sugar levels by avoiding sugar and stimulants and eating slow-releasing carbohydrates such as wholefoods and fruit. Remember that a high-carbohydrate meal can make you drowsy, as can low blood sugar.

Once these basics are handled, and you still need a boost, there are specific supplement recommendations:

▶ 5-HTP: 50mg in the morning, and 50 to 100mg at bedtime to raise your serotonin levels. It is a calming, mood-enhancing amino acid. If you get drowsy from the morning dose, which is very rare, take the entire dose of 50 to 200mg at bedtime.

▶ St John's wort: 300mg of an extract of 0.3 per cent hypericin, starting with one or two capsules/tablets in the morning with breakfast. If there is no change after a week, add a third dose at lunch. You can also take it as two doses of 450mg each, or take your entire daily dose in the morning. If combining with 5-HTP, start with one capsule and build up slowly, since there is the theoretical possibility of serotonin syndrome. This happens when you have an overload of serotonin, and its symptoms are headache, increased body temperature and excessive perspiration. If this should occur, seek medical help as soon as possible.

   You may need a few weeks to feel the full effect. Taking it too close to bedtime can interfere with sleep in some people. Others find it relaxing. Available in tinctures as well, it can be taken in droppersful – just read the label for the dose.

▶ If you tend to be low in energy and unmotivated first thing in the morning, despite sufficient sleep, a 500–1000mg dose of tyrosine or DL-phenylalanine should pick you up. You can gradually increase to 2000mg if necessary.

▶ SAMe is next if you still need a mood boost. Take 200mg twice daily on an empty stomach. If you haven't felt an improvement in a few days, increase gradually, up to 400mg four times daily. Most often, 400mg daily is sufficient. In general, the longer SAMe is used, the more beneficial the results. Once you reach a good level, you can start cutting back to an optimum maintenance dose. Alternatively, take three times as much TMG.

Some mood-enhancing supplement formulas combine these nutrients. The ideal doses are less when combined than when taken in isolation. The following nutrients are worthy additions to a supplement programme designed to elevate your mood.

Mood Enhancers	Combined	Alone
5-HTP	50mg	100mg
St John's wort	300mg	600mg
Tyrosine	500 mg	1000mg
DLPA	500 mg	1000mg
SAMe*	200mg	600mg
TMG	200mg	1000mg
Niacin (B3)	40mg	100mg
Pantothenic acid (B5)	100mg	250mg
Pyridoxine (B6)	20mg	50mg
B12	100mcg	100mcg
Folic acid	100mcg	400mcg

*SAMe does not mix well with other products, so either take it separately or replace it with TMG.

Take the following to lift your mood

▶ A good all-round multivitamin supplying optimal amounts of B vitamins (see 'Natural High Basics', page 33).

▶ **Either** a DHA/EPA rich fish oil supplement **or** fish three times a week in a meal. The fish oils must be taken separately since they are oil and cannot be combined in a tablet.

▶ A mood-booster formula providing many of the nutrients shown above (see Supplement Directory, page 311).

For a full natural mood-lift programme, see 'Top Tips' in Part Four.

MIND AND MEMORY BOOSTERS

W E ALL want to feel sharp and clear-headed – on a real creative roll. A good memory and an active mind will help you generate ideas, solve problems and achieve a terrific feeling of well-being. All too often, however, we feel dull and fuzzy, and have to wrack our brain to pin names to faces, or recall schedules and phone numbers. We don't perform anywhere near our peak.

If your memory isn't as good as it used to be, your concentration flags and you mind feels blunted, you may be another victim of a widespread epidemic: brain drain. You may find that you turn more and more to coffee, sugar and other stimulants in a vain effort to kick-start your mind. But as we saw in Chapter 5, this isn't much of a solution.

You *can* get your mind in gear again – working even better than before, in fact. And we'll show you how. By the end of this chapter you may well feel that feeling on top of the world is within your grasp. But first, let's identify where your problems lie.

The Mind and Memory Check

To see where you fit in the mind and memory continuum, check yourself out on the questionnaire overleaf.

Score 1 for each 'yes' answer.

How Good is Your Memory?	Yes	No
Is your memory deteriorating?	☐	☐
Do you find it hard to concentrate and often get confused?	☐	☐
Do you sometimes meet someone you know quite well but can't remember their name?	☐	☐
Do you often find you can remember things from the past but forget what you did yesterday?	☐	☐
Do you ever forget what day of the week it is?	☐	☐
Do you ever go looking for something and forget what you are looking for?	☐	☐
Do your friends and family think you're getting more forgetful now than you used to be?	☐	☐
Do you find it hard to add up numbers without writing them down?	☐	☐
Do you often experience mental tiredness?	☐	☐
Do you find it hard to concentrate for more than one hour?	☐	☐
Do you often misplace your keys?	☐	☐
Do you frequently repeat yourself?	☐	☐
Do you sometimes forget the point you're trying to make?	☐	☐
Does it take you longer to learn things than it used to?	☐	☐

If your score is:

Below 5: You don't have a major problem with your memory – but you'll find that supplementing natural mind and memory boosters will sharpen you up even more.

5 to 10: Your memory definitely needs a boost – you are starting to suffer from brain drain. Follow all the diet and supplement recommendations in this chapter and check your stress levels.

More than 10: You are experiencing significant memory decline and need to do something about it. As well as following all the diet and supplement recommendations in this chapter, see a nutritionist who can identify other causes of memory decline such as stress hormone imbalances.

You Must Remember This ...

Do you sometimes know you know something but just can't quite make the connections? For example, you know the face but can't remember the name. The reason for this is that memories are held not in one, but in several brain cells joined together in a network. The memory itself is thought to be stored when the structure of a fundamental molecule within brain cells, called RNA, is altered. For a memory to be encoded, it must enter the cells by the mechanism of your seeing, hearing or doing something. This results in three kinds of memory – visual, auditory and kinaesthetic. If you want to be sure you remember something, you need to bring all these into play, and involve the maximum number of brain cells. To remember a telephone number, look at it, repeat it to yourself aloud and punch the numbers on the phone several times. That's the best way to connect.

First, though, we need to take a look at the whole picture – how memory loss is affecting us as we age. Then we'll see what can be done about it. As it happens, there's quite a lot.

The Big Fadeout

In most people, 20 per cent of brain cells die over a lifetime. When you reach seventy your brain will have shrunk by 10 per cent. With this shrinkage often comes a gradual loss of control of the complex orchestra of hormones and neurotransmitters that keep you on the ball. The result is diminished brain power, slower memory retrieval, reduced sex drive, less energy, less motivation and fewer highs. Declining mental function, which often starts to become noticeable in a person's forties, is not inevitable, however, as we'll see.

According to the drugs companies, memory decline is becoming a massive and widespread problem. 'Age-related memory impairment affects many more people than Alzheimer's disease, although, it's certainly true, it is a much less severe condition. We believe at least 4 million people in the UK suffer from this,' says Dr Paul Williams of Glaxo SmithKline, who have been developing drugs to enhance memory and mental performance.

So widespread is the epidemic of age-related memory decline that the pharmaceuticals industry has developed more than 140 types of 'smart' pills in its laboratories, making them the tenth largest class of drugs being researched, according to a report in *The Economist* magazine. Even larger than the market for Alzheimer's is the market for drugs to treat this new problem of 'age-related memory decline'. In much the same way that hyperactivity was only taken seriously once it was classified as a real disease called 'attention deficit disorder', giving a name to this gradual loss of memory will mean doctors can prescribe smart drugs to those whose memories need a boost. As you'll see in this chapter, we recommend smart nutrients – our natural mind and memory boosters – instead.

Even more worrying is the fact that Alzheimer's is on the increase. What could be worse than losing your mind when your body has many years to run? Yet that is precisely what happens to one in ten people over the age of 65, and one in two people over the age of 85. With an ever-ageing population, 20 per cent of the population over 65 will have Alzheimer's by 2030. The stress it brings, both to the sufferer and the family, is immense. For many people on the slippery slope to Alzheimer's, the first signs are depression, irritability, confusion and forgetfulness.

Stress has an enormous impact on our memories, too. A mild dose of stress can actually stimulate memory and mental alertness, but long-term stress is definitely bad news: it puts too much of the hormone cortisol into circulation, and this literally damages the brain. Raised levels of cortisol have been linked to poorer memory and a shrinking of the brain's memory sorting centre.[1] When you were a student, did you stress yourself out revising night after night for exams and then perform badly on test day? The burnout of prolonged stress messes up memory recall.

After only 2 weeks of raised cortisol levels, the dendrite 'arms' of brain cells, which reach out to connect with other brain cells, start to shrivel up, according to research carried out at Stanford University in California by Robert Sapolsky, professor of neuroscience.[2] The good news is that such damage isn't permanent. Stop the stress and the dendrites grow back.

Total Recall: How to Bring It All Back

It all sounds pretty grim. But luckily, you can actually reverse all these trends, from damage by stress to age-related memory loss. Short of a dip in the Fountain of Youth, here's how.

Reduce your level of stress and anxiety, which will in turn cut your cortisol load. Chapter 4 can help here. You need to cut back on stimulants such as tea, coffee or cigarettes and opt for natural alternatives such as ginseng, which halts the overproduction of cortisol, and improves the ability of the adrenal glands to respond to stress (see Chapter 5, page 88).

Take action now. Neither age-related memory loss nor Alzheimer's is inevitable – you can build new brain cells at any age. Research clearly shows that healthy, well-educated elderly people can show no decline in mental function right up to death, and no increased rate of brain shrinkage even after 65. It's a 'use it or lose it' situation. And the steps you need to take to keep all your marbles are the same as those needed to maximise your memory and mental alertness. So, whether you are 20 or 60 years old, the time to act is now.

Eat a diet high in antioxidant nutrients and supplement antioxidant nutrients such as vitamins A, C, E, selenium and zinc (see 'Natural High Basics', page 32). Oxidants damage your brain, and without a good supply of antioxidants, brain cells become more vulnerable to the depredations of free radicals. By the same token, be sure you eat plenty of brain fats. Omega-3 fats from oily fish and flaxseeds and phospholipids, are particularly important (see 'Natural High Basics', pages 29, 30).

Boost your supply of acetylcholine. This neurotransmitter is key to improving memory and mental alertness – people suffering from Alzheimer's, for instance, show a marked deficiency in it. Happily, it's easy to do this by taking choline and DMAE, supplements which we'll discuss in detail below. It's vital to underline, however, that acetylcholine, while it is the major player as far as memory is concerned, is only one of a large cast of neurotransmitters. Some stimulate mental processes, while others calm down information overload. You need the right balance.

It can help to look at the family tree of the neurotransmitter GABA and its cousins glutamate, pyroglutamate and glutamine (see the figure on page 12). The stimulating neurotransmitter glutamate helps forge links between memories, but in some forms too much can literally over-excite neurons to death. This is how the taste enhancer MSG (monosodium glutamate), notoriously used in a lot of Chinese restaurants, turns up the volume on tastes. But too much of it can definitely be a bad thing. On the other hand

GABA, a close relative of glutamate, calms down the nervous system. If you want to enjoy a good memory throughout your life, you have to get the balance of these neurotransmitters right.

And there's more – a range of substances that can give our mind and memory that extra boost. First we'll take a necessarily brief look at what's on offer from the pharmaceuticals companies, then we'll see how we can get that truly *compos mentis* buzz again with natural alternatives.

Smart Drugs and Hormones: A Select Few

With age-related loss of memory on the increase, but a growing need for better mental performance to fit our multi-tasking lifestyles, it's no surprise that a new family of mind-boosters has burst on the scene – the smart drugs. Although they're prescribed for people with diagnosed memory problems, there's a growing underground use of them.

Over a hundred smart drugs have emerged. (For more details see the feature on smart drugs and hormones on www.naturallyhigh.co.uk.) Some block the breakdown of neurotransmitters, some mimic or improve the action of neurotransmitters and some are manufactured versions of hormones that influence brain function, such as melatonin. They are an interesting lot, but for several reasons we don't discuss them here: they're difficult to obtain, some have serious side-effects, and the natural alternatives are very effective. We'll take a look at those now.

Natural Mind and Memory Boosters

If smart drugs are out, what about smart nutrients? There are nine natural mind and memory boosters that can really restore your clarity of thought and banish memory lapses. They are:

▶ Choline and DMAE – the building blocks of acetylcholine
▶ Pyroglutamate, phosphatidyl serine and omega-3 fats – receptor enhancers
▶ Acetyl-L-carnitine and glutamine – fuel for brain cells

▶ Ginkgo biloba and vinpocetine – circulation improvers

▶ Certain vitamins and minerals.

With the exception of ginkgo biloba, these are all substances found in food and the brain. They're becoming widely available, and you can buy combination state-of-the-art brain-boosting supplements in health-food stores, and find them in certain foods. We'll look at each in turn, then discuss why combining smart nutrients works best.

Choline: the building block of memory

The key brain chemical for memory is acetylcholine. A deficiency in it is probably the single most common cause for declining memory. Acetylcholine is derived from the nutrient choline. Fish, especially sardines, are rich in it, hence the old wives' tale of fish being good for the brain. Eggs are also a major source of choline, followed by liver, soya beans, peanuts and other nuts. Ever since egg phobia set in, the average intake of choline from diet has dropped dramatically. From the point of view of memory enhancement, it is certainly worth eating more eggs. Or, if you don't fancy the fat in eggs, you can supplement. But you don't simply make more acetylcholine by eating choline-rich foods – you also need vitamin B5 (pantothenic acid) to form acetylcholine in your body, as well as vitamins B1, B12 and C.

Supplementing choline has some truly remarkable effects. Recent research at Duke University Medical Center, North Carolina, has shown that giving choline during pregnancy creates the equivalent of superbrains in the offspring. The researchers fed pregnant rats choline halfway through their pregnancy. The infant rats whose mothers were given choline had vastly superior brains with more neuronal connections, and consequently, improved learning ability and better memory recall, all of which persisted into old age. This research showed that giving choline helps restructure the brain for improved performance.[3] Based on this study, and numerous others showing the brain-enhancing properties of choline, plus the fact that choline has no known toxicity, supplementing choline in pregnancy is likely to enhance development.

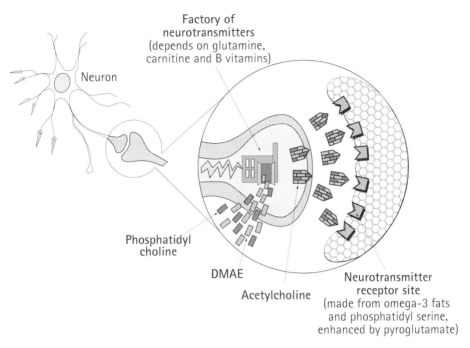

Nutrients that support the memory molecule acetylcholine

Supplementing choline in adults has also proven to boost memory, if given in high doses. For example, Florence Safford of Florida International University gave 41 people aged 50 to 80 choline in 500mg doses every day for 5 weeks. They reported having half as many memory lapses as before, such as forgetting names or losing things. If you combine choline with other smart nutrients such as pyroglutamate, you can achieve the same memory-boosting effect at lower doses (see page 140).

Choline not only makes acetylcholine, the memory neurotransmitter, it is also a vital building material for nerve cells and the receptor sites for neurotransmitters. According to Professor Wurtman from the Massachusetts Institute of Technology (MIT), piracetam and other nootropic drugs (meaning those that boost cognition but are non-toxic) that stimulate the release of acetylcholine should not be given without choline. If your choline levels are depleted, your body grabs the choline that you need to build your nerve cells to make more acetylcholine. So, Wurtman believes, providing the brain with this smart nutrient is essential.

Some forms of choline cross more easily from the blood into the brain. These include phosphatidyl choline and a precursor for choline called DMAE (short for dimethylaminoethanol), which we'll investigate below. Phosphatidyl choline, or PC for short, is also found in lecithin, a supplement widely available in granules or capsules.

Choline

How it works: Precursor for the neurotransmitter acetylcholine and part of structure of neuronal membranes.

Positive effects: More alert, clear-headed, better memory and concentration, improved brain development during pregnancy.

Cautions: None.

How much?: Lecithin 5–10g (tablespoon) or Hi-phosphatidyl choline lecithin 2.5–5g (heaped teaspoon) or phosphatidyl choline 1–2g or choline 300–600mg.

DMAE: let's concentrate

DMAE, like choline, is plentiful in sardines as well as anchovies, but gets from bloodstream to brain cells much faster. Once in the brain it accelerates the production of acetylcholine and reduces anxiety and racing minds, improves concentration and learning, and acts as a mild brain stimulant. It is a great natural mind and memory booster.

The ability of DMAE to tune up your brain was well demonstrated in a German study from 1996 with a group of adults with cognitive problems.[4] The participants had their EEG brain waves measured and were then given either placebos or DMAE. There were no changes in EEG for those on the placebos, but those taking DMAE showed improvements in their brain-wave patterns in those parts of the brain which play an important role in memory, attention and flexibility of thinking.

A variation of DMAE is marketed as the drug Deaner or Deanol, and after numerous trials these have been shown to help people with learning problems, attention deficit disorder and memory and behaviour problems. In one survey by Dr Bernard Rimland from the Autism Research Institute in San Diego, Deaner was found to be almost twice as effective in treating children with ADD than the widely used drug Ritalin, without the side-effects. If you want to boost your memory, the ideal dose of DMAE is 100mg up to 300mg, taken in the morning or midday, not in the evening. Don't expect immediate results: DMAE can take 2 to 3 weeks to work. But it's worth waiting for.

Here's what three people said about their experiences:

I've been taking DMAE for several weeks and I've noticed an amazing difference in mood and concentration level. *AFB, Austin, Texas*

I am currently taking 100mg of DMAE per day and notice a real difference in my alertness, energy level and decreased need for sleep. *RS, Seattle, Washington*

I've been using DMAE with pantothenic acid and a good multivitamin for 2 months now. One of the first things I noticed was that I fall asleep faster and wake up with a clearer mind. I experience a much sounder, more restful sleep. I constantly feel more attuned to my creative potential and I'm always in a good mood. I truly feel alive and awake. *PW*[5]

DMAE

How it works: Precursor for choline which crosses readily into the brain, hence helping to make acetylcholine.

Positive effects: More alert, improves concentration and reduces anxiety, improves learning and attention span, normalises brain-wave patterns.

Cautions: Lower the dose if you find you experience insomnia. Too much can over-stimulate and is therefore not recommended for those diagnosed with schizophrenia, mania and epilepsy.

How much?: 100–300mg, taken in the morning or midday, not in the evening.

Pyroglutamate, PS and omega-3 fats: get receptive

With neurotransmitters, their ability to deliver the message depends on having good 'ears' – that is, fully functioning receptor sites. These receptor sites are built out of two key nutrients – phosphatidyl serine or PS and our old friends, the versatile essential fats, principally the omega-3 fat DHA. The amino acid pyroglutamate, a beneficial form of glutamate, has also been found to vastly improve the brain's ability to receive messages, which in turn promotes learning and memory, by upping the numbers of acetylcholine receptor sites and improving reception.

Pyroglutamate: the master of communication

Pyroglutamate is an amino acid that's key to enhancing memory and mental function. It's highly concentrated in the brain and spinal fluid. So powerful are its effects that there are now many slight variations of this key brain chemical being marketed as nootropic drugs for learning and memory-related problems such as Alzheimer's. Numerous studies using these drugs, one of which is piracetam, have proven that they enhance memory and mental function, not only in people with pronounced memory decline but also in those with so-called normal memory function.[6]

Pyroglutamate does three things that help improve your memory and mental alertness.

▶ It increases acetylcholine production

▶ Boosts the number of receptors for acetylcholine

▶ Improves communication between the left and right hemispheres of the brain.

In other words, it improves the brain's talking, listening and cooperation. It is probably for these reasons that it improves learning, memory, concentration and the speed of reflexes. It can really give you an extra mental edge.

As it's an amino acid, pyroglutamate is found in many foods, including fish, dairy products, fruit and vegetables. Arginine pyroglutamate is the most common form found in straight nutritive supplements. Pyroglutamate is often found in the brain-boosting supplements sold in health-food stores.

Pyroglutamate

How it works: Increases acetylcholine production and improves reception.

Positive effects: Improves memory, cognitive function and concentration, coordination and reaction time, and improves communication between right and left hemispheres of the brain.

Cautions: None.

How much?: 400–1000mg a day.

Phosphatidyl serine (PS): the memory molecule

Known as the memory molecule, phosphatidyl serine can genuinely give some oomph to the brain. It's widely available in health-food stores. PS is a member of the family of phospholipids (see Chapter 3, 'Natural High

Basics'), which are essential for the health of the liver, immune system, nerves and brain. PS is especially plentiful in the brain and there's more and more evidence showing that supplements of it improve memory, mood, stress resistance, learning and concentration. The secret to the memory-boosting properties of PS is probably due to its ability to help brain cells communicate. This is because the 'docking port' for neurotransmitters such as acetylcholine is literally built out of PS.

While the body can make its own PS, we rely on receiving some directly from diet, which makes it a semi-essential nutrient. The trouble is that modern diets are deficient in PS unless you happen to eat a lot of organ meats, in which case you may already be consuming 50mg a day. On a vegetarian diet you're unlikely to get even 10mg a day. So it's probable you'll need to supplement.

PS is particularly helpful for people with learning difficulties or age-related memory decline. In one study, supplementing PS improved the subjects' memories to the level of people 12 years younger. Dr Thomas Crook from the Memory Assessment Clinic in Bethesda, Maryland, in the US, gave 149 people with age-associated memory impairment a daily dose of 300mg of PS or a placebo. When tested after 12 weeks, the ability of those taking PS to match names to faces (a recognised measure of memory and mental function) vastly improved.[7]

Phosphatidyl Serine

How it works: Building material for neuronal membranes and neurotransmitter receptor sites.

Positive effects: Improves mood, memory, stress resistance, learning and concentration.

Cautions: None.

How much?: 100–300mg a day.

Omega-3 fats: why fish is good for the brain

As your grandmother may have told you, fish is good for the brain – especially tuna, mackerel and their oily cousins. She may not have known its mind-boosting power lies in the essential fats it contains. As we've seen already, EPA and DHA, found mainly in oily fish and also in flaxseed, hemp and walnut oils, are omega-3 fats that uniquely feed the brain. (See 'Natural High Basics', page 29.)

DHA, more than EPA, is highly concentrated in our brain and nervous system, making up half of all the fat in brain-cell membranes and improving not only learning and age-related memory but also mood. The higher your blood levels of DHA, the higher your levels of acetylcholine and serotonin are likely to be. The reason for this is that DHA builds receptor sites, as well as improving reception. According to Dr J. R. Hibbelyn, who discovered that fish eaters are less prone to depression, 'It's like building more serotonin factories, instead of just increasing the efficiency of the serotonin you have.'[8]

In one study, people with depression were given 9.6mg of omega-3 oils and experienced substantial improvement in their manic depression over a 4-month period.[9] DHA has also been found to improve dyslexia and dyspraxia. Dr Jaqueline Stordy of the University of Surrey found DHA improves the reading ability and behaviour of adults with dyslexia.[10]

EPA, on the other hand, is proving the more important omega-3 fat in treating schizophrenia. While it is not directly involved in building the receptor sites, EPA makes prostaglandins – information molecules that also tune up the brain and promote healthy brain function. So this fat is more involved in the transmission of information, while DHA is more involved in the reception – all of which is why we need both.

An ideal intake of EPA and DHA is in the order of 500 to 1000mg of each a day, or double if you have one of the mental health problems we've discussed above. (Most fish oils provide about equal amounts of EPA and DHA, so your actual DHA requirement is half this – 250 to 500mg.) Alternatively you can eat 100g of fish – preferably mackerel, herring, sardines, tuna or salmon – three times a week.

BEST FISH FOR BRAIN FATS	AMOUNT OF DHA IN 100G (3½ OZ)
Mackerel	1400mg
Herring	1000mg
Sardines	1000mg
Tuna	900mg
Anchovy	900mg
Salmon	800mg
Trout	500mg

A good-quality cod liver oil supplement can provide up to 400mg of EPA and DHA in total. The most concentrated supplements provide 700mg per capsule. For vegetarians, flaxseed oil is the most direct source of omega-3 fats. In practical terms you need the equivalent of either a level tablespoon of flaxseeds, or a dessertspoon of flaxseed oil, which is also available in capsules. You will need to take quite a few of the capsules to make up the equivalent of the actual oil. Each capsule usually provides 1000mg of the oil, and you need to take eight of these to get the equivalent of a tablespoon of flaxseed oil.

DHA

How it works: Building material for neuronal membranes and neurotransmitter receptor sites, and increases acetylcholine and serotonin levels.

Positive effects: Improves learning, memory and mood in both depression, manic depression, dyslexia and dyspraxia.

Cautions: None. DHA does help reduce blood clotting. High doses should not be taken if you are on blood-thinning medication.

How much?: 250–500mg a day as a fish oil supplement, or eat 100g of oily fish three times a week.

EPA

How it works: Precursor for prostaglandins which influence mood and behaviour and probably neurotransmitter balance.

Positive effects: Helps restore normal behaviour in mental illness. May have effects on mood and memory.

Cautions: None. EPA does help reduce blood clotting. High doses should not be taken if you are on blood-thinning medication.

How much?: 250–500mg a day as a fish oil supplement or eat 100g of oily fish three times a week.

Ginkgo biloba: go with the flow

Ginkgo biloba is a herbal remedy for memory enhancement that's been used in the East for thousands of years. Its first medicinal use can be traced back to 2800 BC, and it comes from one of the oldest species of tree known. Research has shown that it improves short-term[11] and age-related memory loss,[12] slow thinking, depression, circulation and blood flow to the brain. It has also been seen to significantly improve Parkinson's and Alzheimer's diseases within a year.[13] Ginkgo contains two chemicals called ginkgo flavones glycosides and terpene lactones, which are behind its remarkable healing properties.

As well as being a powerful antioxidant, helping vitamin E and other antioxidant nutrients protect your brain from damage, it also helps in the production of neurotransmitters and normalises acetylcholine receptors. However, its major benefit is its ability to improve the circulation of blood in the brain by mildly dilating blood vessels and inhibiting the action of platelet-activating factor, a substance that thickens the blood. So ultimately, ginkgo helps to get oxygen and other important nutrients into the brain.

A review of ten studies testing ginkgo's effects on people with circulation problems, carried out by Jos Kleijnin and Paul Knipschild from the University of Limburg in the Netherlands, found significant improvement in memory, concentration, energy and mood.[14] A more comprehensive double-blind placebo-controlled trial carried out by P. L. Le Bars in France on 18 people aged 60 to 80 found remarkable improvement in the speed of thinking and learning, almost comparable to those of healthy youngsters.[15] Some in the group taking ginkgo were given 320mg, and some 600mg, but both performed nearly as well.

Ginseng seems to fire the action of ginkgo. A recent research study carried out by Professor Wesnes from the University of Northumbria gave 256 healthy volunteers between the ages of 36 and 66 a combination of ginkgo and ginseng, or a placebo. After 14 weeks the people taking the herbal combination performed much better in memory tests. One volunteer said, 'I felt like I was thinking clearer and wasn't so mentally drained at the end of a long stressful day. I noticed I was able to recall things that I had trouble remembering before.'

Ginkgo is usually taken in capsule form and you should look for a brand that shows the flavonoid concentration, which determines strength. The recommended flavonoid concentration is 24 per cent, and you can take two to three doses of 100 to 160mg. Often it takes a month or two before you begin to see results. Ginkgo is a blood-thinning agent so you must use caution if you're taking other blood thinners such as coumadin, heparin or even aspirin. Side-effects of headaches, nausea or nosebleeds have been reported, but only rarely and at high doses.

Ginkgo Biloba

How it works: Improves circulation, acts as an antioxidant.

Positive effects: Improves mood, memory, concentration and energy.

Cautions: Blood thinner: use with caution if already taking blood-thinning medication. Rare side-effects of headaches, nausea or nosebleeds have been reported at high doses.

How much?: 100–160mg a day of a standardised extract providing 24 per cent flavonoids, taken in two or three doses.

Vinpocetine: the secret of the periwinkle

Much like ginkgo, vinpocetine, which is the name for the active ingredient in the periwinkle plant (*Vinca minor*) improves blood flow and circulation, thus helping deliver oxygen to the brain. Research carried out at the University of Surrey gave 203 people with memory problems either a placebo or vinpocetine. Those on the vinpocetine showed a significant improvement in cognitive performance. Research in Russia has also found vinpocetine to be potentially helpful for those with epilepsy.[16]

Vinpocetine

How it works: Improves blood flow and circulation to the brain.

Positive effects: Improves cognitive performance. Potentially helpful in epilepsy.

Cautions: None reported.

How much?: 10–40mg a day.

Vitamins and minerals: a brain's best friend

It's official: multivitamins make you brainier. This was first proven by a research study involving 90 students, carried out by Gwillym Roberts, a schoolteacher and nutritionist from the Institute for Optimum Nutrition, and Dr David Benton, a psychologist from the Department of Psychology at Swansea University College in Wales. A total of 60 students took a special multivitamin and mineral supplement designed to ensure an optimal intake of key nutrients or a placebo, and 30 were given no supplement at all.[17] After 8 months, the IQs of those taking the supplements had risen by over 10 points! No changes were seen in those on the placebos, or a control group of students who had taken neither. More than a dozen similar studies have since been done and, even with lower nutrient doses, smaller but still significant IQ changes have been reported. For example, a study at the University of California gave vitamins and minerals at the recommended dietary allowance (RDA) level and achieved an average increase of 4.4 IQ points. Almost half of the students on supplements had an increase in IQ of 15 or more points.

Exactly how vitamin and mineral supplementation increases IQ scores was worked out by psychologist Wendy Snowden from Reading University's Department of Psychology. In her trial she also gave children supplements or placebos. The children taking supplements showed significant increases in IQ scores after 10 weeks. A close analysis of performance in the IQ tests showed the same error rate, but fewer unanswered questions after the 10 weeks of supplementation. Since almost all the unanswered questions came towards the end of the test, when the children ran out of time, the children on supplements seemed to answer questions faster (hence fewer omissions).[18] This suggests that the effect of the vitamin and mineral supplements was to increase the speed of processing, perhaps by increasing concentration, which clearly a significant factor in intelligence. In other words, vitamins don't increase your inherent intelligence, but they help you to think faster and concentrate for longer.

While few similar studies have been performed on adults, it's highly likely that optimum intakes of vitamins and minerals can improve concentration and speed of information processing in adults. One study carried out by Dr Benton at University College Swansea gave 127 adults ten times the RDA levels of vitamins and minerals, or dummy pills.[19]

After 12 months, the women were showing real improvement in attention and mental performance. Why the men didn't respond remains a mystery.

Of all the vitamins and minerals, B vitamins have the most important roles to play in ensuring optimal brain function because they're vital for delivering oxygen to the brain and protecting it from harmful oxidants. They also turn glucose into energy within brain cells, and help to keep neurotransmitters in circulation. They are, in short, your brain's very best friends. Let's see how they do it.

▶ B3 (niacin) is particularly good at enhancing memory. In one study, a group of subjects of various ages took 141mg of niacin a day. Memory was improved by 10 to 40 per cent in all age groups.[20]

▶ B5 (pantothenic acid) helps improve memory and mental alertness. Sharpen up your memory by taking between 250 and 500mg a day. As we've seen, it's essential for the formation of acetylcholine (see Chapter 2).

▶ B6 (pyridoxine) is a must in making neurotransmitters. It's also necessary for converting amino acids into serotonin – a deficiency in this important neurotransmitter can cause depression and other problems (see Chapter 2). One study showed that about a fifth of depressed people who took part were deficient in pyridoxine.[21] Even 20mg a day can improve your memory, but suggested supplementation is 20 to 100mg a day.

▶ B12 (cyanocobalamin) has been shown in laboratory experiments to speed up the rate at which rats learn.[22] B12 is very important for the health of nerve cells. A loss of these is a prime cause of mental deterioration and confusion in older people. You need 10 to 100mcg of B12 a day. Some people have very poor absorption of B12, and may benefit from much higher amounts, such as 1000mcg daily. Taking B12 in an under-the-tongue formula improves its absorption.

▶ Folic acid, like B12, is essential for oxygen delivery to the brain. A deficiency in either causes anaemia. You need about 400mcg daily.

B Vitamins

How they work: Turn glucose into energy in neurons, co-factors for making neurotransmitters, help transport oxygen, protect the brain from toxins and oxidants.

Positive effects: Raise IQ, improve energy, memory, mood and concentration.

Cautions: None in sensible doses. Excess B3 and B6 can have adverse effects, so don't take more than 1000mg a day. B3 as niacin acts as a vasodilator, improving circulation (and causing blushing) at doses above 50mg.

How much?: For B1, B2, B3 and B6: 50–100mg. For B5: 50–500mg. For B12: 10–1000mcg. For folic acid: 400mcg.

Acetyl-L-carnitine: the brain's superfuel

The amino acid carnitine can be used directly as brain fuel. Acetyl-L-carnitine or ALC is especially useful because the 'acetyl' part helps to make acetylcholine – the key memory neurotransmitter. Supplementing ALC helps to promote both acetylcholine production and release.

ALC also acts as an antioxidant, protecting against brain damage and keeping your nervous system youthful. In animals, it helps to stimulate the growth of new brain cells and improves communication between the right and left hemispheres of the brain.

Plenty of studies have proven ALC's mind- and mood-enhancing properties. You need between 250 and 1500mg for a noticeable effect, and it becomes even more effective if taken with phosphatidyl serine. Unfortunately, it is very expensive and is perhaps not our smart nutrient of choice for this reason. It's best to take it some time before or after eating to maximise absorption.

Acetyl-L-carnitine

How it works: Fuel for the brain, helps make acetylcholine and acts as an antioxidant.

Positive effects: Improves mood and mental performance.

Cautions: Not recommended for those with diabetes or liver or kidney disease.

How much?: 250–1500mg, not with food.

Glutamine: more superfuel

Glutamine, another amino acid, is also used directly as fuel for the brain and has been shown both to enhance mental performance and decrease addictive tendencies.[23] Supplementing glutamine, which the brain uses to build and balance the neurotransmitters GABA and glutamate, can help promote memory. It can be a very useful addition to a supplement programme if you are breaking your addiction to sugar or stimulants (see Chapter 5). We recommend 2 to 5g a day – the equivalent of a teaspoon of glutamine powder, which is much more cost-effective than tablets. It is best not taken with food to maximise absorption.

Glutamine

How it works: Fuel for brain cells, helps build and balance neurotransmitters.

Positive effects: Improves mental energy, reduces addiction, stabilises blood sugar, promotes memory.

Cautions: None. Rare reports of headaches at high doses.

How much?: 2–5g a day, not with food.

Synergy: Together We're Terrific

All these proven mind boosters are remarkable in their own right, but together they rev up your brainpower amazingly. Supplementing smart nutrients such as phosphatidyl choline, pantothenic acid, DMAE and pyroglutamate boosts mind and memory far more in combination than individually. Take the following study. A team of researchers led by

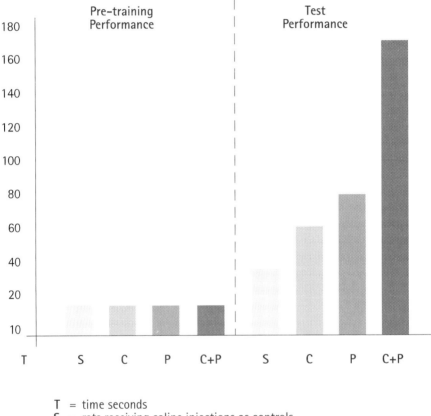

T   = time seconds
S   = rats receiving saline injections as controls
C   = rats receiving choline
P   = rats receiving piracetam
C+P = rats receiving a combination of choline and piracetam

Memory effects of mind-boosting nutrients on
lab rats (see opposite)

Raymond Bartus gave choline and piracetam, a derivative of pyroglutamate (see page 140), either separately or in combination to aged lab rats noted for their age-related memory decline.[24] The team reported that the 'rats given the piracetam/choline combination exhibited memory retention scores several times better than those with piracetam alone'. A study on humans was then carried out by Dr S. Ferris and associates at New York University School of Medicine. These researchers, too, found dramatic clinical improvements, way beyond those given with either choline or piracetam separately.[25]

While both choline and piracetam improved memory, the results showed that half the dose was needed with a choline/piracetam combo. This illustrates the power of combining just two smart nutrients. We recommend combining all the smart nutrients discussed in this chapter for the most effective natural mind and memory boost.

Some smart nutrient supplements contain combinations of all these acetylcholine-friendly nutrients – choline, DMAE, pantothenic acid and pyroglutamate. The ideal doses are less when combined than when a substance is taken alone. If you want to shine mentally and fit names to faces with ease, take the smart nutrients in the table under the Action Plan, in the doses indicated.

Action plan to boost mind and memory

To hone your cognitive abilities and memory, you may need to make some changes in your diet. Here's how.

▶ Eat fish three times a week, with preference for mackerel, herring, sardines, tuna or salmon. Vegetarians need to have a tablespoon of ground flax seeds a day, or a dessertspoon of flaxseed oil.

▶ Supplement a good all-round multivitamin supplying optimal amounts of B vitamins (see 'Natural High Basics', page 33).

▶ Supplement a 'smart nutrient' formula providing the nutrients and amounts shown below (see Supplement Directory, page 311).

▶ Supplement either a DHA/EPA rich fish oil supplement or eat fish three times a week or flaxseeds every day.

▶ Have a dessertspoon of lecithin or a heaped teaspoon of Hi-phosphatidyl choline lecithin a day. (Smart nutrient formulas rarely contain enough phosphatidyl choline because it's bulky.)

If you are over 50 or suffering from age-related memory decline consider adding one or more of the following:

▶ Phosphatidyl serine   100mg
▶ DHA/EPA (fish oil supplement)   500mg
▶ Glutamine (a heaped teaspoon)   5000mg
▶ Acetyl-L-carnitine   1000mg

Smart Nutrient	Combined	Alone
Phosphatidyl choline (PC)	200mg	1000mg
DMAE	200mg	400mg
Pyroglutamate	300mg	700mg
Phosphatidyl serine	50mg	200mg
DHA and EPA*	500mg	1000mg*
Ginkgo	100mg	160mg
Vinpocetine	10mg	40mg
Niacin (B3)	40mg	200mg
Pantothenic acid (B5)	200mg	500mg
Pyridoxine (B6)	20mg	100mg
B12	10mcg	100mcg
Folic acid	200mcg	800mcg

*DHA is an oil and cannot be added to dry supplements.

To sum up, you should take the following

▶ A good all-round multivitamin supplying optimal amounts of B vitamins, vitamin C (see 'Natural High Basics', Chapter 3).

▶ A 'brain-boosting' formula providing phosphatidyl serine, choline, DMAE, pyroglutamate, ginkgo or vinpocetine.

▶ Since most brain-boosting formulas are unlikely to give you enough phospholipids, top them up with a dessertspoon of lecithin or a teaspoonful of hi-phosphatidyl choline on your cereal and a phosphatidyl serine 100mg supplement.

▶ **Either** a DHA/EPA rich fish oil supplement **or** fish three times a week in a meal. The fish oils must be taken separately since they are oil and cannot be combined in a tablet.

For a full, natural mind-enhancement programme, see 'Top Tips' in Part Four.

CONNECTORS

YOU MAY be with close friends, the person you love, or wandering alone in a beautiful place when it hits you: that feeling of being at one with the world. These are experiences that shape and motivate us, and leave us feeling joyful, at peace, part of something bigger than us – in short, connected. We often think of food, clothing and shelter as survival basics, but feeling connected may be the most vital of all.

Of course there are other ways of connecting, such as getting drunk or stoned with friends on a Friday night. But in this case it's not only the company, it's also the chemicals and their inhibition-stripping action that make us feel that sense of connection.

Some of us, sometimes, feel the need for connection far more strongly. We may be going through a bleak patch, or experiencing long periods of isolation, and a sense of not belonging. Then we may begin a search for greater meaning in our lives that can lead to experimenting with 'love drugs' such as Ecstasy or psychedelics such as LSD.

There are big downsides to Ecstasy, LSD and other powerful psychoactive substances, however. You can be let down with a crash, develop tolerance and psychological addiction, or worse. We'll look at the problems in detail, as well as why happiness depends on feeling connected. Then we'll show how certain natural herbs and nutrients help you feel part of it all, not apart. You'll even find ways of blissing out, opening the mind to new frontiers, by simply calling up the brain's own pharmacopoeia. Only connect – and get safely high!

Connection Check

Before we explore these, check out how 'connected' you feel using the questionnaire below.

Score 1 for each 'yes' answer.

How Connected Are You?	Yes	No
Do you lack enthusiasm?	☐	☐
Do you feel lonely much of the time or find it difficult to be alone?	☐	☐
Do you lack good friends you can really talk to?	☐	☐
Are you unclear about your spiritual values?	☐	☐
Do you lack a sense of peace and contentment?	☐	☐
Do you find it difficult to receive love from others?	☐	☐
Do you rarely have experiences of great joy or love?	☐	☐
Do you feel different, like the 'odd one out'?	☐	☐
Do you lack a sense of purpose or meaning in your life?	☐	☐
Do you rarely feel a connection with nature?	☐	☐
Do you lack a sense of self-worth?	☐	☐
Do you abuse your body with bad diet, drugs, overwork or lack of rest?	☐	☐
Do you feel disconnected from your local community?	☐	☐
Do you rarely have peak or transcendent experiences where everything falls into place?	☐	☐

If your score is:

Below 5: You are doing well. You have a better than average sense of purpose and connection in your life. Following the advice in this chapter will help you feel even more connected and perhaps show you the way to peak or transcendent experiences.

5 to 10: This area of your life needs your attention. Consider taking up group activities that promote the sense of connection such as yoga, t'ai chi or meditation classes. Also follow the diet and supplement recommendations in this chapter.

More than 10: You are experiencing a high degree of dis-connection, and need to re-evaluate your life and what is important for you. Have you ever considered seeing a counsellor or psychotherapist or attending a personal development course (see Resources, page 308). Consider taking up group activities that promote the sense of connection such as yoga, t'ai chi or meditation classes. Also follow all the diet and supplement recommendations in this chapter.

The Chemistry of Connection

Feeling good about yourself, and connected to others, has a lot to do with our mental and spiritual health. But it's also down to chemistry. We've seen how a lack of GABA makes you stressed, a lack of dopamine makes you unmotivated, how serotonin deficiency leaves you depressed, how insufficient acetylcholine leads to mental exhaustion. A big part of feeling connected is having every one of these neurotransmitters in balance – to be firing on all cylinders.

So, the best opening strategy for feeling connected and happy is to learn how to fine-tune the balance of your neurotransmitters through diet, supplements and lifestyle changes, as we've outlined so far. The energy and well-being this will give you will be the perfect springboard for greater things, as we'll see.

Peak Experiences: The Bigger Picture

Once you feel happy and good about yourself, and sure of your place in the world, that can be wonderful – for a while. But then there is that basic human urge for meaning, to know what life is all about. Some of us can begin to feel complacent. And that's where a quest for transcendent or 'peak' experiences can begin. By transcendent we mean a greater sense of unity or harmony, a real connection with others and a profound sense of purpose in life. These are the flashes of inspiration that often fuel great works of music, art and poetry, as well as scientific and spiritual breakthroughs.

By their very nature peak experiences are very hard to put into words. Patrick remembers having such an experience while meditating.

The meaning in life is the slightest shift like driving a car round the corner into a panoramic view or breaking through fathoms of dim water into the light. Nothing is different, nothing is the same. What once was your life, is now only a game. Like breathing air for the very first time, it feels so natural, it feels so right to be bathing in this radiant light.

The experience gave him a whole new perspective on various problems he was grappling with at the time.

Most of us have already had peak experiences. Perhaps you were deeply in love, or had a profound, life-changing insight. You may have felt a flash of the 'bigger picture', or of the connectedness of everything, when you were in the midst of stunning natural beauty. You may even have experienced a spiritual awakening through meditation or another discipline – or had a drug-induced mind-altering experience. And it's these we're going to look at now – the psychoactive drugs known as 'entheogens', or 'substances that take you towards unity'. Ecstasy (MDMA), psilocybin mushrooms and LSD all belong to this class of drugs.

Take Jerome's experience. This 70-year-old retired engineer from the US took Ecstasy legally in 1980, under the guidance of a psychotherapist:

> Before, I had thought of reality as being just the concrete reality that we see before us. MDMA made me see other, generally invisible realities, almost visions, that co-exist with it. I could see the interconnnectedness of all people and all things, and felt a powerful love emanating from within me. I saw my partner in a totally different way – with absolute acceptance and love. It was an exquisite dance of harmony and pure love. I became a happier, more fulfilled person, more complete in many ways. It has coloured my life ever since.

It's not surprising that young people out in the world, away from their first source of connection – the family – have embraced Ecstasy. In the UK an estimated half a million Ecstasy tablets are taken every week, mainly by 16- to 25-year-olds. The figures for people older than this show that use of such substances usually falls away or becomes much rarer.

Without meaning to condone the use of MDMA – there are considerable downsides, discussed on page 166 – the fact that a chemical can, under certain circumstances, help to induce a life-changing, transcendent experience warrants investigation. In our search for natural highs we want to know what's going on in the brain during peak experiences, whether chemically induced or not, and discover the natural ways to bliss out without the downsides.

We'll be looking at 40 years of research into the chemistry of connection. The study of how entheogens alter consciousness has led to discoveries that can open doors to a natural high. But first, some background.

Plato Took Acid: The History of Getting High

In case you think the use of entheogens is a minority activity of little relevance to humanity's quest for natural highs, take a look at history. Virtually every culture through history has used these substances. In India almost 4,000 years ago, the Vedas – Hindu philosophical texts – extol a plant potion called *soma*, considered to be God in plant form. The ancient Greeks, from Aristotle to Plato, took part in an initiation called the Eleusian mysteries that involved consuming a rye-based drink. Historians believe this contained the ergot-rye fungus, a natural source of LSD. Egyptian cultures used the blue lily, henbane and mandrake, which were also favourites of European witches.

In the Americas, the Mayans discovered that certain mushrooms, and the skin of certain toads, contained powerful hallucinogens. Some Native American tribes use the peyote cactus to this day. Probably the earliest use of 'magic' mushrooms predates even this, back to the Siberian peoples of north-east Asia who later crossed the Bering Strait to colonise the Americas. They revered the highly toxic *Amanita muscaria*, or fly agaric, a red and white spotted mushroom. To this day a herbal brew known as yage or ayahuasca is still used widely by South American shamans.

In the West, the mostly widely used entheogens are 'designer drugs', manufactured compounds such as Ecstasy and LSD.

Expand your mind: how entheogens work

Our brains filter out the vast majority of information that comes in through our senses. This allows us to make sense of the world and also has survival value. Our awareness seems to work much like a lighthouse, always scanning for potential danger in one or another spot. We see what we need to see for our survival. And this is a mere fraction of what is actually out there.

When an entheogen is taken, this filter is suspended. The person under the influence is seeing the bigger picture. It sounds amazing, and as we've seen in Jerome's story, it is. But there are dangerous downsides to entheogens: many of them are extremely toxic and the experiences aren't always good. We'll go into these below, but first let's see precisely how entheogens dissolve the filter in our brains. This will give us some vital clues to finding the best natural connectors.

DMT: key to connection

In the vast majority of entheogens, the active compounds are substances called tryptamines. These are chemical cousins of a key brain chemical, di-methyl tryptamine (DMT), which is closely related to the 'happy' neurotransmitter serotonin. (Ecstasy is slightly different, as it also has a major effect on dopamine, the 'feel-good' neurotransmitter.)

DMT acts much like a neurotransmitter, and is a mind-expanding substance in its own right thought to be produced primarily in the pineal gland, along with serotonin and melatonin. The pineal, which is at the centre of the brain, is light sensitive in many animals. Therefore, it is necessary for them to be connected to the environment and the ebb and flow of day and night, as well as seasonal changes. The Indian mystics consider it our 'third eye', an antenna, if you like, for inner light. (Have you ever thought where the light comes from when you dream?) René Descartes also considered the pineal gland to be the seat of the soul. As you can see in the figure overleaf, entheogens all have profound effects on the neurotransmitter serotonin and, perhaps most importantly, on DMT.

As we've seen, substances that stimulate the release of or mimic the effects of a neurotransmitter generally lead to downregulation. In other words, you get the high, followed by the low. This is exactly what happens with most entheogens: you don't feel so good the next day. Also, the more often you take them, the weaker the effect. For example, many people who take Ecstasy report that its effect diminishes the more often it's taken.

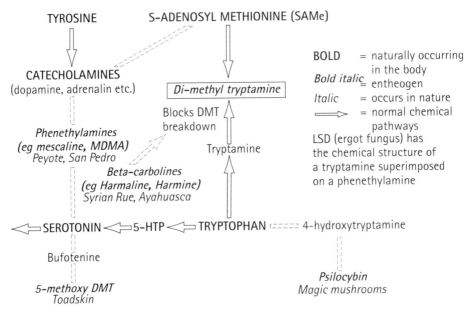

The family tree of entheogens

But just like the neurotransmitters dopamine, serotonin or acetylcholine, DMT works every time. This suggests that we all have within us the chemistry that is associated with expanded awareness and feeling connected, *all the time.*

Of course, most of us *don't* feel permanently connected. Why not? Perhaps it's partly because we don't make enough DMT, or our brains rapidly break down the DMT we produce. If you inject DMT into the bloodstream, it produces an immediate change in consciousness, but because it's broken down quickly the effect doesn't last that long. There is some evidence that people with certain types of schizophrenia may excrete more DMT in their urine, indicating they may have an excess of it. So, too much isn't such a great idea either. Here again, it's a question of balance.

We have a long way to go in uncovering the chemistry of consciousness, but it looks like neurotransmitter activity, as an overall pattern, is involved in the action of our brains' selective filters. If your neurotransmitters are out of balance, perhaps because you're too stressed or depressed, or not getting enough of the right nutrients, you don't hear the 'full orchestra', so to speak. But when the filters are suspended, we hear the whole symphony of life. As William Blake said, 'If the doors of perception were cleansed everything would appear to man as it is: Infinite.'

How much exposure to infinity can we stand, though? Is it always a good thing to have mind-altering experiences? And if so, are there downsides to using entheogens such as Ecstasy or LSD to get there? And are there natural connectors, with no downsides? These are the questions we explore next.

Ecstasy, LSD and Magic Mushrooms: What Goes Up ...

There are hundreds of entheogens to be found in nature, and hundreds more man-made designer drugs. Most of these are rarely used and are of little interest to us here. (For further information, see *The Encyclopaedia of Pyschoactive Substances* – details on page 303 – and www.maps.org.) The most commonly used are Ecstasy, psilocybin or 'magic' mushrooms and LSD, and it's their downsides we'll investigate here. But first, a look at the pitfalls of all entheogens:

▶ **Tolerance**. The more often a person takes entheogens the less their effect becomes. This phenomenon is almost certainly a consequence of overstimulating the neurotransmitter pathways, which in turn leads to both depletion of the neurotransmitter in question and downregulation (see Chapter 2). Tolerance is a major problem with Ecstasy.

▶ **Coming down**. For the same reasons, when the effects of taking an entheogen wear off, most people feel disconnected, possibly depressed, and tired. Despite this they may be unable to sleep because depleted serotonin can cause insomnia.

▶ **Addiction**. Entheogens are not physically addictive in the way that cocaine or heroin are. They can, however, be psychologically addictive – the person can crave a repeat of the experience. Often, as the thrill from taking the drug wears thin with time, a person will take more of it.

▶ **Bad trips**. Most entheogens present a very challenging psychological experience. It's not at all uncommon for someone to become extremely anxious and fearful in the face of what is essentially a shock to his or her normal reality. The result – a 'bad trip'. If you are at all unstable, an experience like this could leave you very fragile emotionally or even precipitate you into mental illness, so think twice before taking an entheogen. Far from experiencing a sense of connection, you may end up feeling extremely alienated from what you're feeling and the people you're with.

Psilocybin mushrooms: how magic are they?

Psilocybin is the major psychoactive agent in so-called 'magic' mushrooms (*Psilocybe cubensis*). This is one of many tryptamine-containing fungi that have been used for thousands of years throughout Europe, Asia and the Americas.

Depending on dosage, the effects of taking them include:

▶ Nervousness
▶ Nausea
▶ Greater emotional sensitivity
▶ Visual hallucinations
▶ Time distortions.

As with most entheogens, when the effects wear off there is a feeling of fogginess and tiredness, though sleep doesn't always come easily. Occasionally, very high doses cause vomiting, although the mushrooms are not very toxic. Other species of psychoactive mushrooms, such as *Amanita muscaria* or fly agaric, can be extremely toxic and even fatal.

LSD: the acid test

Lysergic acid diethylamide, abbreviated to LSD, was discovered in 1938 by Albert Hoffman working for the Sandoz pharmaceuticals company. It became a drug of choice in the 1960s and 1970s, popularised by celebrities such as Dr Timothy Leary of 'Turn on, tune in, drop out' fame. LSD, one of the most powerful entheogens, is produced from ergotamine, which is found in fungi that typically grow on rye. A related compound, ergonovine, is found in several species of morning glory seeds. The amount needed to produce an effect is tiny compared to other entheogens.

LSD was used extensively in psychotherapy during the 1960s, but, for some people the experience is far from positive. Effects can include:

▶ Visual hallucinations
▶ Time distortions
▶ Over-awareness and over-sensitivity to music and noise
▶ Paranoia
▶ Fear and panic
▶ Unwanted, overwhelming feelings
▶ Flashbacks (see below).

Physically, you may experience:

▶ Jaw tension
▶ Sweating
▶ Nausea
▶ Dizziness
▶ Impaired coordination and judgement.

An LSD experience is called a 'trip' because it is much like a journey to another place. And as we've indicated, this can be a very confronting experience. Oscar Janiger, who pioneered research into LSD back in the 1950s, interviewing hundreds of people after LSD trips, came to this conclusion.[1]

LSD seems to produce a marked shift in our fundamental perceptual frame of reference, upon which rests our ongoing concept of reality. This change in our habitual way of being in the world may lead to a profound psychic shake-up and may provide startling insights into the nature of reality and into how our personal existence is fashioned.

As we've seen, however, LSD can result in extreme fear. It can be very dangerous if you are:

▶ Unstable or immature
▶ Have a strong attachment to your ego
▶ Have a pre-existing deep-seated emotional trauma
▶ Suffer from mental illness.

Despite its Class A status (a category reserved for drugs considered to be most harmful when misused), LSD isn't actually physiologically addictive, nor has it been found to damage the brain. Like other tryptamines, it raises the release of serotonin which is followed by serotonin depletion. This makes it harder to sleep, so, the day after a trip, the person can feel tired and subdued. It is relatively non-toxic, perhaps because the dose needed is so small, and has no known lethal dose.

So the main risk from taking LSD is psychological trauma. LSD's notorious flashbacks are related to this. Strong negative experiences while under the influence of LSD can be strongly imprinted in your memory, and when these memories are triggered later the initial experience may be relived to a degree.

Agonising over Ecstasy

Can it cause brain damage?

Long touted as relatively safe, Ecstasy is looking increasingly dangerous after numerous research studies. While the jury is out on whether LSD and psilocybin damage the brain, concerns about Ecstasy started to be raised when studies on animals, carried out in the 1980s, showed damage to neurons.[2] Following on from this research, Dr George Ricaurte of Johns Hopkins University in Baltimore and Professor Una McCann of the US National Institute of Mental Health near Washington DC gave monkeys a 4-day course of Ecstasy. A fortnight later, they killed part of the test sample and looked at their brains. For Ecstasy, or MDMA, to qualify as neurotoxic in their study, there had to be damage remaining after 2 weeks. There was.

Seven years later, the researchers killed the remaining monkeys to find out whether the monkeys' bodies could repair MDMA-induced brain damage once it was incurred. There was still damage. 'Clearly, the amount of MDMA is important, but it's also important to recognise that even a single dose of MDMA may be enough to produce neuro-injury,' concluded Dr Ricaurte.[3]

It can be argued that this study was done, not on Ecstasy-popping clubbers, but on primates, and at high doses. There is still room for uncertainty about its effects on humans. But the study does prove that MDMA can cause irreversible brain damage.

Worries over long-term brain damage have been further fuelled by research published in the *Lancet* in 1998.[4] Brain scans of heavy Ecstasy users showed damage to serotonin neurons caused, they believe, by MDMA. Such damage would be likely to promote a tendency to depression and poor mental function. This study involved subjects who reported taking Ecstasy in high doses more than 200 times in less than five years. Their average dose – 386mg – was also exceptionally high. However, it is difficult to believe that Ecstasy was the only drug used in high doses by these subjects, so it is not possible to conclude that all the damage to serotonin neurons was caused by MDMA, or that infrequent use causes the same kind of damage.

Not all studies have shown damage, and it certainly appears that damage is very dose-dependent. However, the weight of the evidence to date tends to point in the same direction. It suggests that MDMA can damage neurons, specifically serotonin receptors, and lead to serotonin deficiency. (For a thorough discussion of the research, please see 'The Politics of MDMA research' by Dr Charles Grob, reprinted on our website www.naturallyhigh.co.uk.)

Can it be deadly?

Deaths from Ecstasy use have been reported in the media, even of first-time users. According to the UK's Police Foundation, who made a thorough evaluation of risk, 'Although deaths from Ecstasy are highly publicised, it probably kills fewer than ten people each year, which, though deeply distressing for the surviving relatives and friends, is a small percentage of the many thousands of people who use it each week.' It's not always clear what killed these unfortunate few, although the vast majority of deaths are caused by dehydration. This is because people on Ecstasy dance for hours and are too high to realise they need to drink water to replace lost fluids and cool down. More than half of all Ecstasy-related deaths also involve other drugs, the most common being alcohol. So far, there is no clear case of death actually caused directly by MDMA, except for the case of an unfortunate dog that died shortly after being given a massive amount of MDMA.[5]

Having said that, very high doses of MDMA in some people may cause serotonin overload, which can be fatal. This suggests it would be exceedingly unwise to take MDMA with an anti-depressant drug that blocks the breakdown of serotonin.

Are there aftershocks?

Some people have few, if any, significant after-effects from taking Ecstasy. According to Dr Una McCann, who carried out important research on MDMA with Dr George Ricaurte:

> This makes people think it's safe. I think the danger is people are slowly damaging their brains and are totally unaware of it. I think the older they get, they [users] will be much more vulnerable to a variety of problems such as depression, memory disturbances, anxiety disorders and sleep difficulties.[6]

Whether or not this is true is still a bone of contention, but the evidence is clearly pointing towards memory problems with long-term MDMA use. The more you use it the more you lose it

A review of seven studies published in the last 10 years came to the following conclusion:

> There is enough evidence to think that heavy MDMA use may cause medium to long-term disruption in short-term memory and/or some types of mental function. The data so far is too weak to say for certain whether this is true or what percentage of users would be affected. The changes are subtle and are more

likely the more frequent the use, the higher the dose, and/or the larger the lifetime total use. The data is far from conclusive, but certainly suggested caution for those who use MDMA regularly or heavily.[7]

Ecstasy has been described as 'the new beer', yet as the numbers who use it rise, more and more cases of adverse after-effects are coming to light. Depression and paranoia are the most commonly reported, memory loss less so. Consider Tahnia's story.

A few months after starting taking Ecstasy I noticed I wasn't getting so high. I had to have more, two tablets instead of one, to get the sense of joy I experienced at the beginning. The more I took the more depressed I became. I was feeling more afraid, more lost and increasingly more unhinged. One night I took a double dose and had awful hallucinations. I was depressed all the next week, crying a lot and unable to communicate with anybody, even my boyfriend. It was after this experience that I realised that the drug I had taken to lift me to new highs had actually sent me far lower than I had experienced before taking it. I quit.

Tahnia's experience highlights the dangers. Today's club scene encourages the frequent recreational use of MDMA and other drugs, such as 'cocktails' containing methamphetamine. Coupled with lack of sleep and poor nutrition, this combination can increase the sense of unreality, and MDMA's cumulative effects can send some users over the edge.

Like Tahnia, many people report that their enjoyment of MDMA seems to decrease every time they take it. Some users report that E 'loses its magic' with as few as ten experiences. Most voluntarily stop taking it because they experience an actual increase in negative side-effects such as depression and 'hangovers', as well as poorer highs. So far, there has been very little research into other reported concerns, including risks of cardiac arrhythmias, hypertension, strokes and adverse drug interactions of MDMA.[8] But it needs to happen.

The final verdict? Magic mushrooms, LSD and Ecstasy are illegal. And because they are illegal there is no quality control, so you may be taking something far more toxic than you expect. It's a fake paradise at best, a short-cut to achieving a temporary experience of enhanced perception and a state of connection. At worst, taking man-made drugs such as MDMA frequently and in combination with other drugs leaves you vulnerable to potentially irreversible brain damage.

As depressing as all this sounds, we can definitely take you higher. We'll now take a look at how – via completely natural nutrients and herbal connectors.

Natural Connectors: Be At One

You know those times when you feel completely in tune with others and the world seems a wonderful place? No, it isn't a Fred Astaire song – and, it isn't the world that changes: it's the way you see it. And the way you see it is affected by both your brain's chemistry and your frame of mind. Entheogens such as Ecstasy can temporarily get you 'high', but at a cost. Natural connectors, on the other hand, combined with lifestyle changes that help develop the right frame of mind, can help you to feel connected most of the time, with no downside in sight.

We'll be investigating a handful of natural connectors that are widely available in health-food stores:

▶ Tryptophan or 5-hydroxytryptophan
▶ S-adenosyl methionine (SAMe) and tri-methyl glycine (TMG)
▶ B3, B6, B12 and folic acid
▶ Kava
▶ Sceletium.

The chemistry of connection is all about having a healthy balance of neurotransmitters, specifically dopamine, serotonin and DMT. The best way to achieve this is to supplement a cocktail of supporting nutrients. The figure opposite shows how these promote a healthy balance of DMT and serotonin.

Here's what happened to Jeremy, a psychologist who decided to try natural connectors.

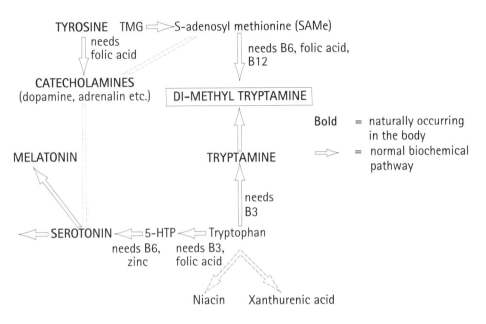

How natural connectors promote a healthy balance of DMT and serotonin

My life had become a rollercoaster of highs and lows, with many more lows than
highs. I decided to clean up my act for a month, and started taking 5-HTP, SAMe
and B vitamins, plus kava in the evenings. Within a week I stopped feeling like a
'victim' and started to feel in charge and in tune and my mood and outlook on life
noticeably improved.

As you can see above, the building block of both serotonin and DMT is
the amino acid tryptophan, an essential constituent of protein. In addition,
the brain's chemistry is carefully and intelligently kept in order by catalysts
that have the ability to change tryptophan into a number of natural
connectors. These catalysts are SAMe, and the B vitamins that add or
remove what are known as 'methyl' groups. (DMT, the brain's natural
connector, is a type of tryptamine with two methyl groups added, hence
the 'di-methyl'.) It has long been known that a deficiency in these nutrients
can induce schizophrenia – the profound 'dis-connection' of a person.
These combinations of nutrients therefore help to fine-tune brain
chemistry, to allow for a more natural and consistent state of connection.

Tryptophan and 5-hydroxytryptophan: crucial connectors

The amino acid tryptophan, a normal constituent of food, is the basic building block not only of serotonin, but also of tryptamines, such as DMT. As such, tryptophan is critical to the chemistry of connection. As already discussed (see Chapter 6), tryptophan deficiency leads to depression, while supplementing tryptophan has proven an effective antidepressant.

As far as promoting a natural state of connection is concerned the objective is to make sure that the brain and nervous system have an adequate supply of this vital amino acid. This not only depends on your daily intake of tryptophan, but also your intake of B vitamins.

Unfortunately tryptophan is only available in the UK on prescription, as an antidepressant called Optimax by Merck. This was banned for over-the-counter sale following the distribution of a contaminated batch produced by a Japanese manufacturer, which resulted in an outbreak of the serious disease, eosinophilia myalgia syndrome. A number of people died in what was the first major blunder of genetic engineering – the manufacturer had genetically modified an organism to produce tryptophan.

Tryptophan itself is, however, both safe and effective. Since it competes for absorption with other amino acids, its absorption is assisted by ingesting carbohydrate which helps carry tryptophan from the blood into the brain. So if you are taking Optimax, have it with a fruit snack, and avoid eating proteins an hour before or after.

Tryptophan

How it works: Indirect precursor for the neurotransmitter serotonin, DMT and all tryptamines. Can be converted into niacin (vitamin B3).

Positive effects: Improves mood, promotes healthy sleep-wake patterns and emotional stability, dreaming and visioning. An effective antidepressant.

Cautions: None reported, but it's inadvisable to take both tryptophan and SSRI antidepressants except under medical guidance.

How much?: 1000–3000mg for the treatment of depression or insomnia, 1000mg as a natural connector. Best absorbed away from food or with a carbohydrate snack, such as a piece of fruit. If used for insomnia, take 1 hour before bedtime. Best taken with B vitamins.

5-HTP: 'Hawaii in a bottle'

More effective and more readily available than tryptophan, 5-HTP (5-hydroxytryptophan) is a more biologically active form of it. While 5-HTP is not a direct precursor for DMT, it is the most effective precursor for serotonin (see the figure on page 171). By providing the brain with the raw material to make serotonin this spares tryptophan for producing other important tryptamines, such as DMT.

Described by one magazine as 'Hawaii in a bottle', 5-HTP can have profound mood-lifting effects. Here's what happened to Alex after he took 5-HTP.

I had recently ended a long-term relationship and often felt lonely and a bit down, missing that company and connection. On good days I felt fine, looking forward and getting on with life, but they were few and far between. I started supplementing 200mg of 5-HTP a day. Within a couple of days I felt much more 'up', in the moment and basically happier. I had more of an enjoyable, warm sense of detachment, that everything was all right, rather than a kind of gloomy seriousness. I don't take it all the time but when I've 'lost the plot' I include this in my daily supplement regime.

5-HTP is ten times more powerful than tryptophan, so the dose needed for a psychoactive effect is a tenth. Like tryptophan it has proven to be at least as effective as the best antidepressant drugs, but without the same high risk of side-effects (see Chapter 6). 5-HTP occurs naturally in an African plant, *Griffonia simplifica*, and is available as a nutritional supplement.

Because 5-HTP doesn't compete for absorption with other amino acids, it is well absorbed both with food and without. The amount needed to promote a sense of connection is 100mg a day, or less if taken in combination with other 'connecting' nutrients.

A word of caution: more is not better. Within 2 hours of serotonin overload, 'serotonin syndrome' can trigger frightening symptoms: tremor, nausea, vomiting, elevated temperature, abnormal heartbeat. Except in extreme cases, where it can be fatal, symptoms will subside within 6 to 24 hours. Serotonin syndrome does not occur with either tryptophan or 5-HTP in anything close to the dose ranges we recommend. However, we do not recommend simultaneously supplementing these nutrients with antidepressant drugs, which effectively keep more serotonin in circulation by stopping its breakdown, unless under medical guidance. Nor do we recommend combining these nutrients with entheogens such as Ecstasy and LSD that temporarily raise serotonin levels

5-Hydroxytryptophan (5-HTP)

How it works: Direct precursor for the neurotransmitter serotonin.

Positive effects: Improves mood, promotes healthy sleep-wake patterns and emotional stability, dreaming and visioning. An effective antidepressant.

Cautions: Some people report nausea, anxiety and agitation at very high levels. It is inadvisable to take both 5-HTP and SSRI antidepressants except under medical guidance.

How much?: 100–300mg for the treatment of depression or insomnia, 100mg as a natural connector. If used for insomnia, take 1 hour before bedtime.

S-adenosyl methionine (SAMe): the master tuner

As far as the chemistry of connection is concerned, SAMe (pronounced 'Sammy') is the master tuner. The body can and does make SAMe from the constituent of protein, methionine. Having enough vitamin B6, B12 and folic acid helps the body maximise its production of SAMe. As you can see in the figure on page 171 it donates 'methyl' groups and helps to make naturally occurring tryptamines – part of the brain's well-tuned chemistry. The methylation of tryptamine, for example, results in DMT.

SAMe also helps neurotransmitters deliver their messages to the receptor sites by sharpening up their activity. By methylating phospholipids, from which nerve cell membranes are made, SAMe improves cellular communication between nerve cells.

SAMe can also help you get a good night's sleep, and promotes dreaming. This is because the brain's manufacture of melatonin, a key neurotransmitter for sleep and dreaming, from serotonin, depends on SAMe.

Although SAMe has been proven to be an antidepressant,[9] it can enhance a feeling of well-being and connection. While a positive response is often felt within a week, and often within days, it may take as long as 4 weeks. In general, the longer SAMe is used, the more beneficial the results.

SAMe should be taken on an empty stomach, preferably 1 hour away from food. Start with a dosage of 200mg twice daily. If results aren't seen in a few days, you can gradually increase it, up to a maximum of 400mg four times daily, if needed. Most often, 400mg per day is sufficient. SAMe should also be taken with its co-factors, vitamins B6 (100mg) and B12 (100mcg), and folic acid (1000mcg). It is safe to use during pregnancy and breast-feeding.

Pharmaceutical-grade SAMe comes in two forms, tosylate and a newer, more stable form, called butanedisulfonate. The former quickly degrades upon exposure to heat and/or moisture. However, both forms are relatively stable in enteric-coated tablets, which means that they aren't destroyed by stomach acid and release the SAMe lower in the digestive tract. They also reduce the chances of nausea and gastrointestinal disturbances. Reducing the dose size and taking it with meals usually overcomes this potential problem, although this will also somewhat reduce its potency.

Unfortunately, SAMe is relatively expensive. In comparing products, potency and price, look for the amount of active ingredient on the label. For example, 200mg of s-adenosyl-methionine butanedisulfonate provides only 50 per cent or 100mg of SAMe. Purchase from a reputable company, not one newly on the SAMe bandwagon.

A word of caution. Higher doses may lead to irritability and anxiety. If this continues even on the lowest dose, stop taking SAMe. There are no reported negative interactions with other medications or nutritional supplements. In manic-depressive patients, SAMe can even trigger a manic episode (as can any antidepressant).

S-adenosyl methionine (SAMe)

How it works: Catalyst for producing a wide range of key brain chemicals, including DMT, serotonin, dopamine and noradrenalin. It works by donating a 'methyl' group, and thereby helping to synthesise key brain chemicals. It is itself produced from the amino acid methionine. Also important in detoxifying the liver.

Positive effects: Acts as a stimulant for well-being. Generally improves energy, mental clarity, emotional balance and mood, promoting natural connection.

Cautions: In some people higher doses of SAMe have been known to induce nausea. It is therefore better to start low with 200mg and work up. Taking SAMe with food reduces this possibility, but reduces the overall effect.

How much?: 400mg up to 1000mg on an empty stomach, which helps absorption.

Trimethylglycine (TMG): the SAMe again

Until less expensive SAMe supplements become widely available, your best bet is to supplement trimethylglycine (TMG). The body can make SAMe directly from TMG, which is both stable and much less expensive. While it has not been so extensively researched as SAMe, the fact that it is a direct precursor of SAMe would predict that its effect would be very similar although you need more. Also, TMG helps the body to make more SAMe from dietary protein.

TMG is extracted from sugar beet and is also found in broccoli and spinach. It has no reported side-effects other than brief muscle tension headaches if it is taken in very large quantities without food. Optimal doses needed to raise SAMe levels in the body are 1000 to 3000mg per day. A 500mg dose is sufficient enough in a combined formula.

Trimethylglycine (TMG)

How it works: Precursor for SAMe (see above).

Positive effects: Acts as a well-being stimulant. Generally improves energy, mental clarity, emotional balance and mood, promoting natural connection.

Cautions: Very high doses can cause headaches.

How much?: 500–3000mg a day. Best absorbed on an empty stomach.

B3, B6, B12 and folic acid: a brain's best friends

If SAMe is the source of the methyl groups that transform one brain chemical into another, B vitamins are the delivery boys who can accept or donate methyl (carbon-based molecules) groups. They are the real workers in the enzymes that turn one brain chemical into another and keep you feeling connected.

For some enzymes you need vitamin B3, for others B6, B12 or folic acid. Not surprisingly, deficiency of any one of these leads to dis-connection, and is associated with depression, mental illness, schizophrenia and unpleasant hallucinations. Supplementing these has the reverse effect, and has been shown to dramatically improve a person's mental and emotional well-being.

As long ago as 1957, Dr Humphrey Osmond and Dr Abram Hoffer, the Director of Psychiatric Research for Saskatchewan, Canada, proved that supplementing niacin normalised behaviour in those diagnosed with schizophrenia in the first ever double-blind study in the history of psychiatry.[10] Dr Hoffer, who is now in his eighties, has treated over 5,000 patients with schizophrenia and claims an 80 per cent success rate using B3 and other connector nutrients. (His definition of cure: free of symptoms, and able to socialise and pay income tax!) Hoffer and Osmond were among the first scientists to investigate the chemistry of entheogens (Osmond introduced Aldous Huxley to mescaline, the entheogen found in the peyote cactus. To describe his experience he wrote *The Doors of Perception*, from which Jim Morrison named his band, the Doors – an interesting connection.) Using this research they developed their theories on how to treat the mentally ill suffering from unpleasant hallucinations. These have proven correct, and to this day Hoffer believes an optimal intake of these nutrients is essential to be naturally high.

Meanwhile, Dr Carl Pfeiffer at the Brain Bio Center in Princeton had also been investigating the chemistry of the brain in relation to mental health and illness. He discovered that a deficiency in vitamin B6, or pyridoxine, and zinc (pyridoxine is 'activated' in the body by a zinc-dependent enzyme) also created dis-connection, diagnosed as mental illness. Supplementing vitamin B6 and zinc corrected this abnormal chemistry and improved their mental health and experience of connection.[11] B6 is now known to help SAMe donate its methyl groups in the chemistry of connection.

Folic acid is also a methyl donor. Research at King's College Hospital and the Institute of Psychiatry in London found that a third of all patients with either severe depression or schizophrenia were deficient in folic acid.[12]

Supplementing folic acid for six months made a big difference in their symptoms and ability to relate.

However, you don't have to suffer from schizophrenia to benefit from these B vitamins. Optimal amounts of these vital nutrients help to keep you well tuned and naturally high. Folic acid, together with vitamin B12, is needed to turn the amino acids tryptophan into serotonin and tyrosine into dopamine to keep you feeling happy and motivated. Without these vitamins the higher brain centres simply can't work at their peak.

Of course, the effect of these nutrients in isolation is not nearly as powerful as they are in combination, and consequently, to enhance connection, it is best to supplement the following levels every day:

▶ Niacin (B3)   100mg
▶ Pyridoxine (B6)   50mg
▶ Cyanocobalamin (B12)   50mcg
▶ Folic acid   400mcg

Plus the minerals . . .

▶ Zinc   15mg
▶ Manganese   5mg
▶ Magnesium   350mg

Niacin comes in two forms – niacin and niacinamide. At doses above 50mg, niacin makes you blush. This effect is beneficial in many ways, but it's not to everyone's liking. To avoid the flushing effect, supplement no more than 50mg of niacin, and take the rest as niacinamide.

B Vitamins

How they work: Co-factors for making neurotransmitters, vital for enzymes that control the chemistry of connection, methyl group donors and acceptors.

Positive effects: Improve energy, memory, mood, concentration, and enhance connection. Prevent unpleasant hallucinations.

Cautions: None in sensible doses. Excess B3 and B6 can have adverse effects (above 1000mg a day). B3 as niacin acts as a vasodilator, improving circulation and causing blushing at doses above 50mg.

How much?: Niacin (B3) 100mg; pyridoxine (B6) 50mg; cyanocobalamin (B12) 50mcg; folic acid 400mcg.

Kava as connector

While we have extolled the virtues of kava as a stress-buster and natural relaxant in Chapter 4, from Hawaii to Papua New Guinea kava has been at the core of life for centuries, as a wonderful connector. Taking kava opens you to an experience of heightened awareness and empathy, of enhanced 'being' and freedom from 'doing'. Traditionally, the feel-good staple of the South Sea islands has two main uses: first, a personal experience of peace, relaxation, ease, well-being, even euphoria; and secondly, a social context, often with a sense of ritual or ceremony. In fact, in Fiji, the phrase 'drinking kava alone' is a euphemistic way of accusing a person of practising black magic!

Kava certainly qualifies as a natural connector. When you take kava, at least in the manner and doses used regularly in the South Pacific, your consciousness is unmistakably altered. It's difficult to improve on the description of anthropologist, E. M. Lemert, who observed:

The head is affected pleasantly; you feel friendly, not beer sentimental; you cannot hate with kava in you. Kava quiets the mind; the world gains no new colour or rose tint; it fits in its place and in one easily understandable whole.[13]

Referring to its subtlety, islanders say: 'Kava doesn't come to you. You go to kava.' Terrence McNally's description of his experience of kava well explains its role as a natural connector:

> Over the next several minutes, at least four things seem to happen fairly simultaneously. A wave of relaxation rolls through my body. The effects of kava are immediate, but they are not abrupt. The second thing is an emotional release, perhaps even more subtle than the physical. I don't notice the change as it happens, but I find I'm feeling at ease, comfortable in my skin, but again very awake.
>
> Vision and hearing are slightly heightened. I've read of the islanders' wanting silence and darkness because of increased sensitivity, but I've never found it uncomfortable. Both sights and sounds are just a little brighter, clearer and warmer. Finally I'm aware of a feeling of easy connectedness and relationship with others in the room.[14]

The potency of kava preparations varies, and the herb affects different people differently. For some, kava's effects are too subtle; for others, too strong. Some people feel no effects the first couple of times they try kava. Others report feeling weird or dopey at first, but experience a clearer, more pleasant state with subsequent use. Kava is most potent when consumed on an empty stomach.

As we've noted, Pacific islanders speak of 'listening to kava'. It opens a window on to subtle awareness and a connection to nature, as well as to others and to oneself. Kava's first effects are felt within half an hour, and its mild high lasts 2 or 3 hours.

Kava has properties that clearly qualify it as an entheogen – increasing feelings of sociability, friendliness and empathy with others. But kava would hardly be described as an hallucinogen. At most, some report that high doses of potent kava can cause mild visual and auditory distortions, such as objects taking on a subtle glow or a softness of focus.

You have to take relatively large amounts of the whole root to feel its mind-altering effects. One serving of the traditional beverage, usually 115 to 170ml (4 to 6 fl oz), contains about 1000mg of resin giving 250 to 500mg of kavalactones. Islanders might consume five or more such servings in a single night. Tablets or capsules would be an unwieldy means for achieving such dosages. While it could be done with tinctures, the most sensible method would be ground kava powder, available in bulk at some herbal outlets or ethnic markets.

Kava definitely affects consciousness and thinking. In studies, memory actually seems to be enhanced. Perception is a bit heightened, and so is sensitivity to stimuli such as noises or bright lights. Unlike alcohol, with kava you're likely to experience no loss of mental sharpness. (In some studies kava actually enhanced it.) But don't be fooled. Kava can deeply relax muscles, almost to the point of numbness. You can still function, but coordination is impaired.

Definitely do not drive, operate heavy machinery, or care for an infant under the too-relaxing influence of kava. Other than this there appears to be no downside to using kava as a connector.

Kava

How it works: Appears to enhance activity of GABA, the relaxing neurotransmitter that also modulates dopamine, adrenalin and noradrenalin. There is still much that is unknown about its effects on the brain.

Positive effects: Heightened sensory perception, relaxation, well-being, connection, empathy. An effective anti-anxiety agent. Also promotes good sleep. A muscle relaxant.

Cautions: Do not drive or operate heavy machinery after use; do not mix with alcohol, as the two substances seem to potentiate each other; do not take while using benzodiazepine tranquillisers.

How much?: As a relaxant, the normal dosage is approximately 75mg of kavalactones; as a connector, 150–500mg (start at the lower dose).

Sceletium: South African gem

According to Dr Nigel Gericke, from the African Natural Health organisation in South Africa:

> Sceletium is one of the most ancient of mind-altering substances, and it is likely to have had a profound influence on the evolution of human consciousness. People interested in consciousness will find that sceletium is a key, but it needs to be used wisely. It is not a quick-fix, and after ten years of use I'm still learning about it.

He is currently spearheading research into sceletium at the University of Natal's department of botany.

An unfamiliar herb to most of us, this native South African creeper, also called kougoed, has been used by hunter-gatherer tribes since prehistoric times. It lessens anxiety, stress and tension, raises spirits and enhances the sense of connection. If you take a very large dose you may even feel euphoric, then taken over by a sense of drowsiness. It does not cause hallucinations. Nor do nearly 400 years of documented use reveal many serious adverse effects, either.

Traditionally, sceletium is chewed, brewed as a tea, or used as snuff. If enough is chewed, it has a mild anaesthetic effect in the mouth, as does kava if chewed, and is used by the San people of South Africa for tooth extractions, or is given in minute doses to children with colic. A tea made from sceletium is used to wean alcoholics off their tipple. In this way the recovering alcoholic can avoid withdrawal symptoms.

People have reported that sceletium-induced relaxation has helped them to focus on inner thoughts and feelings, or to have a heightened experience of the beauty of nature. Some have reported an increased sensitivity of the skin as well as sexual arousal, while others have said it leaves them feeling free of fear and stress. Lewis Lewin, in his 1934 book *Phantastica*, reports that mesembrine – one of the active chemicals in the plant – can induce a meditative state of mind.

While no clinical trials have been published yet, a number of doctors and psychiatrists have reported a wide range of positive uses for sceletium, from treating anxiety and depression to alleviating alcohol, cocaine and nicotine addiction. Moreover, by promoting a sense of empathy and connection, it has also been reported to help couples in therapy.

How does it work? The active constituents of the plant are alkaloids, including mesembrine, mesembrone, mesembrenol and tortuosamine. According to laboratory studies sponsored by the National Institute of Mental Health near Washington DC, its major alkaloid, mesembrine, acts as a serotonin-uptake inhibitor.[15] Like Prozac, it helps to keep more serotonin in circulation. It also appears to have a harmonising and balancing effect on the other feel-good neurotransmitters, dopamine and noradrenalin, as well as on adrenalin.

An effective dose is 50mg a day, although some doctors report needing to use 100 to 200mg a day for those with chronic depression or anxiety.

Sceletium

How it works: Appears to enhance serotonin activity, the mood-enhancing neurotransmitter, and balance dopamine, adrenalin and noradrenalin; there is still much that is unknown about its effects on the brain.

Positive effects: Relieves depression, tension and anxiety, promotes a sense of connection. Associated with insights, heightened sensory perception and improving meditation. Also reduces addictive craving.

Cautions: In very large doses can have euphoric effects, followed by sedation. No reported toxicity.

How much?: As a mood enhancer, the normal dosage is 50–100mg; as a connector, 100–200mg.

Alex, 28, is a new advocate of sceletium.

I used to drink on Friday nights to unwind after my stressful week. Now I prefer sceletium. I combine 100mg of sceletium with 400mg of kava and 1g of TMG. This not only chills me out but it makes me feel very connected and 'present' and able to really enjoy my friends' company. It's a bit like the buzz you get sitting on the beach watching the waves rolling in. What's more, there's no hangover.

Action Plan for Getting Connected

The first steps to feeling connected naturally is to tune up all your neurotransmitters, in other words, follow all the advice so far. This includes reducing your stress level, balancing your blood sugar and reducing your intake of stimulants to an absolute minimum. A good all-round multivitamin is key. Part Three, 'Living High Naturally' also gives you plenty of exercises and lifestyle changes that will promote your sense of connection.

The ideal doses of the 'connector nutrients' are less when combined than when a substance is taken in isolation. The following nutrients are worthy additions to a supplement programme designed to enhance connection. This combination, taken every day, is likely to improve meditation, dreaming, insights and understanding, as well as your mood and ability to relate.

Natural Connector	Combined	Alone
5-HTP*	50mg	200mg
SAMe†	400–1600 mg	–
Or TMG	600mg	1800mg
Kava (standardised extract)‡	100mg	250mg
Sceletium	100mg	200mg
Niacin (B3)	100mg	500mg
Pyridoxine (B6)	50mg	100mg
Cyanocobalamin (B12)	50mcg	100mcg
Folic acid	400mcg	800mcg

*Do not supplement 5-HTP with antidepressant medication. One supplies the precursor to make serotonin. The other prevents the breakdown of serotonin. Taking both could lead to serotonin overload.

†SAMe is best taken on its own. For combination formulas it can be substituted by its precursor, TMG, which is more stable and less expensive, in which case you need triple the dose (see page 177 for more details).

‡The kava dosage given here relates to the actual amount of kavalactones in the product, be it powder, capsules or tincture.

The combination of these nutrients promotes a sense of heightened awareness and connection that far surpasses any individual ingredient. Andrew, a nutritionist, who helped research the effects of this combination of nutrients, is a case in point. Here's what he said:

> There is no doubt that there is an enhanced state. It isn't the quick hit of a drink but there is a definite calming effect which builds almost imperceptibly and with no loss of function. After a couple of drinks I'm normally fading badly within an hour – these nutrients didn't do that to me. It gave a sense of well-being, the relaxing effect of a weak alcoholic drink without the associated dilution of control. A quietly expanded state which is gentle but powerful. I'm still feeling on an up (yet relaxed!) 18 hours later and there is an unequivocal improvement in acuity, perception, enthusiasm, creativity and productivity. Today has been a very good day and it is no coincidence!

To sum up, you should take the following

▶ A good all-round multivitamin supplying optimal amounts of B vitamins (see 'Natural High Basics', page 33), and the minerals zinc, manganese and magnesium.

▶ A 'connector nutrient' formula providing 5-HTP, TMG, kava, sceletium and additional B vitamins to achieve the levels shown above. SAMe is unstable, needs to be refrigerated and supplemented away from food, and for these reasons is often supplemented separately.

For a full natural programme promoting feelings of connection, see 'Top Tips' in Part Four.

PART THREE

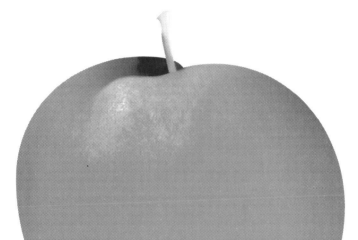

LIVING HIGH
NATURALLY

9

BALANCING THE EQUATION

IN THE last part we described how to influence your balance of neurotransmitters with natural supplements. We should not forget, however, that we actually manufacture our own neurotransmitters. While caffeine can stimulate us, it is doing it though its effects on our brain's own dopamine. Similarly, while Valium or kava can relax us, what's really doing the job is our very own GABA. We also produce our own morphine-like substance, the endorphins, which relieve pain, enhance immunity and make us feel euphoric.

Here we introduce you to other key aspects of the natural high equation that help you to balance your own neurotransmitters and stay high naturally, introducing you to techniques and lifestyle changes that will help to keep you relaxed, alert, productive and happy. We'll be looking at each of the following and giving you specific exercises to try out:

▶ The Exercise High
▶ The Breath of Life
▶ Generating Vital Energy
▶ Meditation and the Mind
▶ The Benefits of Biofeedback
▶ Positive Mental Programming
▶ The Power of Touch
▶ Sexual Chemistry
▶ Light and Colour
▶ Aromatherapy – Healing Scents
▶ The Music of the Emotions
▶ How to Get a Good Night's Sleep

By understanding and incorporating these into your lifestyle, you will learn how to self-regulate your mental and emotional state. Kai's story is a case in point.

I (Hyla) recently ran into Kai, a 23-year-old who had come to me a year earlier for counselling. At the time, he'd complained of moodiness, learning difficulties and not having friends. He admitted to smoking too much marijuana and drinking too much beer. This now exuberant and healthy-looking young man brought me up to date. A month or so on the prescribed supplements had calmed his mind, elevated his mood and energy, and curbed his addictions. I had given him DL-phenylalanine, tyrosine and glutamine, 500mg of each twice daily, plus a high vitamin B multivitamin/mineral formula and 200 to 400mg of Siberian ginseng daily. He also took kava, 70mg twice daily, with more if he felt nervous.

Once he felt stable on this regime, Kai went on to discover his own route to getting high: a meditation technique learned from a spiritual teacher. He not only meditated daily, but managed to incorporate the principles into his daily life. As an example, he recounted his preparations to go to a reggae concert with his buddies (yes, he now had lots of friends). They were all smoking dope to put themselves in the mood. Kai, on the other hand, described how he 'just sat quietly, closed my eyes, looked upward, and soon was in a state of bliss. I was high all the way there, and during the whole show. I didn't have those old problems coming down, either. You know, the low blood sugar, and feeling bad. I can make my own high, and it's an even better one. It's free and legal, too!'

He was rightly proud of his accomplishment. And I was delighted to see his transformation.

Like Kai, you can produce your own natural high. The next section will give you many different ways to activate your own neurotransmitters, from having a positive attitude, to breathing techniques, meditation, exercise and music. Many of these help you to experience the present moment or, in the words of Ram Dass, to 'Be here now'. Much of what ails us and prevents us from being fully happy is being stuck in the past, or racing towards the future. On the other hand, if you can recognise that the past is history, the future is a mystery, and the only time that exists is the present, which is a gift (that's why it's called the present), then you're on the right track for staying high naturally.

Present and Relaxed

While we have to relearn this skill, babies and young children manage to be in the moment with no effort. In fact, so does your cat. Cats and babies don't think about paying the rent, getting to the dentist on time or staying in relationships. They are just there (or 'here'). How can we achieve this state? You can actually do it at a traffic light, in the queue at the bank or while waiting for your lunch date to arrive. You can turn impatience into presence. Use a breathing technique, a meditation as Kai did, or listen to certain music. There are many ways, described in the chapters which follow, that help to bring you back to the present moment.

An integral part of being present is relaxation. This is not the sloppy relaxation of flopping in front of the TV, but a release of tension that is accompanied by a conscious awareness. There are many ways to relax this way:

▶ You can take a deep breath, let it go, and come back to yourself. Instead of worrying about what is not happening, allow yourself to be exactly where you are. You'll find that time will shift, stand still, and you will feel alive, connected and energised.

▶ You can take a quiet walk on the beach, in a park, or in any special place where you can let go of your worries. Enjoy a beautiful sunset. Nature can be the best 'awakener', as we sink into her rhythm, which is ultimately our own. Sometimes, even reminiscing about a pleasant experience in your past will bring you into a happier connection with 'now'.

▶ There are more structured forms of relaxation therapy, as well. Exercise, movement, breathing exercises, yoga, meditation, biofeedback, self-hypnosis, t'ai chi, can all help you approach life with a greater sense of inner calm and expansiveness. It takes only 10 to 15 minutes a day to see results. It often helps to do these techniques in a group: aside from the fun of social contact, the group energy seems to prime the pump, making it easier to reach an altered, relaxed state.

In each of the following chapters, we will describe an activity, how it helps us to be naturally high, and provide a simple exercise for you at the end. You will soon see that the common theme that runs throughout is the state of being fully aware and in the present. You allow all of your senses to come into play – sight, sound, taste, touch, movement, whether you are involved in meditation, deep breathing, exercising, dancing, massaging or being massaged, listening to music, inhaling aromatic oils or making love. Enjoy them. They are free, legal and not fattening!

10

EXERCISE

> ... we need only to disappear in the dance to liberate the sexual, creative, and sacred aspects of the soul ... Energy moves in waves. Waves move in patterns. Patterns move in rhythms. A human being is just that, energy, waves, patterns, rhythms. Nothing more. Nothing less. A dance.
>
> Gabrielle Roth, *Sweat Your Prayers*

(HYLA) was recently hiking in the hills near my home, experiencing the combination of exertion, breathing fresh air and being in nature. Grinning uncontrollably from ear to ear, I arrived home exhausted and totally exhilarated. I realised how I had missed this old familiar feeling. Remember how you felt as a child, running and playing with your whole being – body, mind and spirit? We adults can still recapture some of that same exhilaration with a variety of activities.

We are already aware of the physical benefits of exercise: weight control, and conditioning of heart, lungs, flexibility, bones and muscles. But exercise can also improve our mood by producing positive changes in body and brain chemistry. Exercise not only reduces the release of adrenal stress hormones, but it also increases the supply of blood and oxygen to the brain, and stimulates the release of powerful, mood-elevating endorphins. These chemical messengers create euphoria and pain relief, often hundreds of times stronger than that produced by morphine. This natural 'opium' produces the sensation known as 'runner's high', which even has an addictive quality. Deprived of their 'fix', grounded runners will often become irritable and depressed, much like a junkie withdrawing from heroin.

Oliver, a 43-year-old musician, says 'I used to be into all kinds of stimulants including cocaine.' Now, he says, 'I have discovered running, and I have a clear and consistent high. I feel terrific most of the time, without the lows I used to have after coke. I would not trade this feeling for anything.' Oliver is not alone.

The Endorphin Connection

There have been over a hundred clinical studies examining the link between endorphins and exercise. One of the most interesting was conducted by Dr Dennis Lobstein at the University of New Mexico. He compared ten sedentary men with ten men of similar age who jogged. The sedentary men turned out to be more depressed and with lower levels of endorphins. They also had higher levels of both the stress hormones and of the perceived levels of stress in their lives. Other studies have since established that exercise can be as effective as an antidepressant or traditional psychotherapy in treating low moods.

However, you don't have to be either depressed or a seasoned athlete to benefit from endorphins. Moreover, the more intensely you exercise, the more of these chemicals you produce, and the higher you get. Exercise can also increase self-esteem, as tangible evidence of your desire and to take charge of your life and to improve yourself.

Invitation to the Dance

Dancing to music is one of the most powerful ways to release endorphins. One of the pioneers of dance as a natural high is Gabrielle Roth, whose music is now used in many dance classes. 'I feel my soul in my body when I dance,' writes Gabrielle Roth in her fascinating book, *Sweat Your Prayers*. She describes the night she discovered this.

I got up and started moving, holding nothing back, nothing at all. Lost in the spirit of the dance, I found a path, a dancing path, that took me to the deepest most alive place I had ever seen . . . It was as if I were plugged into the master current and life was charging through me, creating a clarity that I had never known before.

Find music such as hers that will make you dance to your depths, like there is no tomorrow. Sweat a little – it's good for you. You won't be able to stop smiling. Notice variations in mood and tempo, from flowing to staccato, and from chaos to lyrical, as you explore your body and soul in motion. Some 20 minutes a day, and you are reconnected with yourself. (See Resources on page 308 for details and also on page 246 for information about her music.)

'Exercise' Exercise

▶ Whatever form of exercise you choose, it's easier if you do it with a friend. Besides the company it provides, this partnering keeps you committed.

▶ If you have never exercised before, and especially if you have a pre-existing health condition, see your doctor before you begin.

▶ Then, start your exercise programme gradually, such as with a walk around the block.

▶ Build up over time to a slow jog, first around the block, or a track, slowly increasing the distance and speed.

▶ For maximum benefit, build up to a full jog that lasts between 20 and 30 minutes, 4 to 6 days a week.

▶ Jogging, cycling, swimming and calisthenics are all forms of aerobic exercise, which conditions the heart and lungs, and includes dancing, discussed above.

▶ Weight lifting is an example of resistance exercise, which builds your muscles. It also counters osteoporosis, since bone development is stimulated by weight-bearing exercise, and helps to burn fat. Both types of exercise are important to overall health.

▶ All exercise takes your mind off your worries: think of the times when you played tag, football, netball or rounders with your friends. Be a kid again!

▶ Ride your bike, rollerblade, or use an exercise bike while watching a video or reading a book.

If you do this 5 days a week, you will feel fabulous, and look good, too. No matter what activities you choose, keep the following tips in mind:

▶ Wear loose, comfortable clothing and well-fitting running shoes.

▶ Warm up before exercise, use a lot of stretches and cool down afterwards.

▶ Do not fall into the 'pain is good' trap. Some muscular soreness or tightness is normal, but pain is a sign that something's wrong. If the pain persists, stop exercising and see your health practitioner.

▶ Don't overdo it, especially at the beginning. Rest between exercise sessions. Excessive exercise actually evokes the stress response.

▶ Do something you enjoy. The more you enjoy an exercise, the more likely you are to stick with it.

11

THE BREATH OF LIFE

YOU CAN get high on breathing – feel calm, happy and at ease. In fact, there's a whole science of breathing, originating in India called *pranayama*. More on this later. But first, let's look at how what you breathe makes a difference.

Oxygen itself is a natural high. In fact, as we've seen, we make energy in the body from 'burning' carbohydrate with oxygen. Oxygen is really the most important 'nutrient' of all – it makes up about 80 per cent of the human body. After all, if you don't get enough you're dead in minutes.

The assumption is that we all get enough oxygen from breathing. But there's a big difference between good air and bad air. Just compare how you feel when breathing refreshing mountain air, and when choking on polluted city air. The reason you're coughing is down to the impure kinds of oxygen, called oxides, that are found in smoggy air.

Pure oxygen's healing powers are so great that critically ill people are sometimes put in oxygen tents. Within complementary medicine there is a whole speciality, known as oxygen therapy, devoted to ways of enhancing oxygen balance in the body, which has been proven to increase energy and mental alertness. However, there are things you can do right now to increase your ability to use oxygen.

While you might not fancy living in an oxygen tent, the truth is that most of us use less than one-third of our lungs' capacity. Exercise and breathing exercises will help you to maximise your use of lung capacity, thereby helping to oxygenate the tissues and improve your energy and alertness. The best forms of exercise in this respect are aerobic, stamina-building exercises such as swimming, jogging, exercise classes, cycling and brisk walking, which all require you to breathe deeper and harder. Deep breathing is beneficial in all forms of exercise. It is good, when you exercise, to pay attention to your breath and synchronise your movements with your breath as this will help you to breathe deeply, allowing more air in. Exercising in this way is a natural high, promoting energy, exhilaration and a natural connection as your mind and body become 'in sync'.

The Breath of Life

Breathing is something we take for granted. Yet, for thousands of years in India, people have practised breathing exercises called *pranayama* to evoke conscious and healthful changes in the body and mind as a means to natural bliss. Your breathing is a reflection of your emotions.

Each emotional state has its own distinct breathing pattern. For example, when you are anxious or afraid, your breathing becomes rapid and shallow. When you are happy and at ease your breathing is naturally slow and deep. Working with the breath is a fundamental part of meditation and yoga. The breath is said to be the link between mind and body – the key to calming the mind and relaxing the body and promoting a natural high. Conscious breathing is a vital part of a natural relaxation programme.

You can try this yourself right now. Bring to mind something you are stressed or anxious about. Put it to one side for a minute, and focus on your breath. Let your inhalation become a little deeper and your exhalation a little longer. Take nine slow breaths like this, and it's amazing how focusing on your breath can help you become more 'detached' from the emotional charge and help you gain perspective on difficult situations.

In the philosophy underpinning yoga, the air we breathe contains not just oxygen but also *prana*, or vital energy. By practising conscious breathing exercises we can accumulate this energy and revitalise the body and mind.

Science is ever closer to measuring this invisible energy. Some scientists think it's connected with charged particles in the air called ions. When these particles are negatively charged they have positive effects on us, and vice versa. This is what ionisers are all about – they generate negative ions. High levels of positive ions (the bad guys), are found during certain kinds of strong winds, such as the mistral in France or the furn in Switzerland, which are rumoured to make you grumpy and irritable. After a thunderstorm, or close to a waterfall, the air is charged with negative ions – the good guys. These may literally help us to accumulate vital energy.

Unless you happen to have a waterfall close by, another way of doing this is with specific breathing exercises. Most yoga and meditation techniques (see Chapters 12 and 13) teach specific ways to deepen your breathing. This is not only good for oxygen delivery, but also a great way to calm the emotions and clear the mind. Deepening the breathing reduces tension. Dia-Kath breathing, described below and overleaf, is specifically designed to generate this *prana*, the natural, vital energy available to all of us.

Always be conscious of your breath and learn how to breathe deeply to give yourself a natural energy boost, and keep yourself relaxed and clearheaded. Spend as much time as you can in clean air. If you are a city-dweller, choose holidays in the mountains or by the ocean and go for walks in the country.

Breathing Exercise

This breathing exercise (reproduced with the kind permission of the Arica Institute, a school for self-knowledge), connects the *kath* point – the body's centre of equilibrium – with the diaphragm muscle so that deep breathing becomes natural and effortless. You can practise this exercise at any time, while sitting, standing or lying down, and for as long as you like. You can also do it unobtrusively during moments of stress. It is an excellent natural relaxant and energy booster, helping you to feel more connected and in tune.

The diaphragm is a dome-shaped muscle attached to the bottom of the rib cage. The *kath* is not an anatomical point like the navel, but is located in the lower belly, about three finger-widths below the navel. When you remember this point, you become aware of your entire body.

In Dia-Kath breathing, your lower belly expands from the *kath* point as you inhale. The diaphragm muscle expands downwards as if pulled by the *kath* point. This allows the lungs to fill with air from the bottom to the top. As you exhale, the belly and the diaphragm muscle relax, allowing the lungs to empty from top to bottom. Inhale and exhale through your nose.

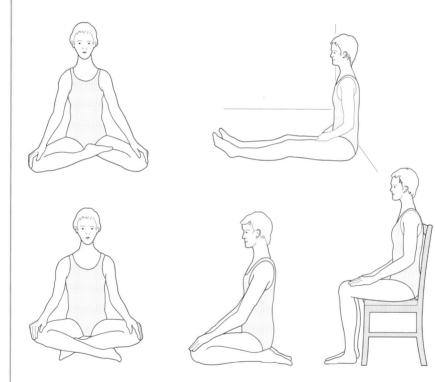

Dia-Kath breathing positions

1. Sit comfortably, in a quiet place with your spine straight, in any one of the positions above.
2. Focus your attention on your *kath* point.

3. Let your belly expand from the *kath* point as you inhale slowly, deeply and effortlessly. Feel your diaphragm being pulled down towards the *kath* point as your lungs fill with air from the bottom to the top. On the exhale, relax both your belly and your diaphragm, emptying your lungs from top to bottom.
4. Repeat at your own pace.

▶ **Every morning sit down in a quiet place** before breakfast and practise Dia-Kath breathing for a few minutes. Breathing in this way can lead you into meditation (see Chapter 13).

▶ **Whenever you are stressed throughout the day check your breathing**. Practise Dia-Kath breathing for nine breaths. This is great to do before an important meeting, or when something has upset you.

Progressive Relaxation

Another breathing exercise is called the *progressive relaxation* response. This is especially good when you need to de-stress and unwind. Lie down and take several deep breaths. Then, breathe in slowly as you tense the muscles in your foot. Hold your breath, and the tension, for a count of 20. (If you don't make it to 20 at the beginning, don't worry.) At 20, slowly breathe out, releasing the muscles until they are totally relaxed. Repeat the process with your calf muscles, and work your way up, finishing with your facial muscles. Close with a few more deep breaths.

12

GENERATING VITAL ENERGY

ENERGY ISN'T just about the food you eat and the air you breathe. It's also dependent on the state of your body. Without exercise, the body loses muscle tone and it accumulates tension – and you feel tired. Exercise improves the circulation and oxygenates the blood, which is a natural high in itself, increasing your energy level. But there's more to exercise than simple physical training and the endorphin effect explained in Chapter 10. Scientific research into yoga and t'ai chi have found health benefits you don't get from aerobics classes or running around the park. While excessive 'aerobic' exercise can actually depress the immune system and overstress the body, t'ai chi can boost well-being and immunity. Yoga has been shown to have positive effects on pulse, blood pressure, and mental and physical performance beyond that expected from physical exercise alone.[1]

These ancient systems of exercise were never designed simply to get you fit. They were designed to generate a natural high by removing the blockages that accumulated tension builds up. Such blockages prevent vital energy – known in China as *chi*, and in India as *prana* – from restoring your vitality.

And we accumulate stress every day, which is stored as anxiety in our minds and as tension in our bodies. In the underlying philosophy of Far Eastern martial arts and the ancient Indian traditions, yoga or t'ai chi unlock the tension and allow you to return to a natural and blissful state of equilibrium.

Yoga: Free Yourself

Relaxation, clarity of mind and energy: practising yoga can give you this. The word 'yoga' comes from the Sanskrit for 'union'. Its origins can be traced back over thousands of years to the very foundation of Indian civilisation. In its truest form yoga is the science and practice of obtaining freedom and liberation. The physical exercises of hatha yoga are only one type of the discipline, in which breath, movement and posture are harmonised to remove physical blocks and tension in the body. As emotional tension is also stored in the body, the aim of hatha yoga is to promote physical, emotional, mental *and* spiritual well-being.

Hatha yoga is itself subdivided into other types, such as iyengar yoga, which is a slower and more precise form using a series of postures to help realign the body so the vital energy can flow properly. Astanga yoga, on the other hand, is a more athletic and physically demanding type of yoga. Both forms will leave you feeling more relaxed and energised, but some people naturally prefer astanga yoga, while others respond best to iyengar. Try them both and see what suits you.

Yoga classes are now widely available (see Resources on page 309). Attending classes regularly is a wonderful way to get naturally high, as Simon's story illustrates. Simon was a vice-president for a record company, with a very busy life and a lot of stress. He tried many alternative approaches, but yoga was what made the biggest difference.

'When I started doing yoga I experienced a sustained energy release that lasted all day. I got into a routine of doing a yoga session almost every day. As well as giving me more energy, I feel much more positive, and how I react to stress has changed. Things that used to bother me before and cause me stress now don't cause me anything like the same degree of agitation. Practising yoga hasn't made me slow down as such. I'm still very busy but I'm much calmer about everything.'

Simon found the benefits of yoga so great that he now teaches it at the Triyoga Centre in London.

Once you've learnt the postures, you can practice yoga at home, perhaps accompanied by a video or some relaxing music.

T'ai Chi: Movement in Meditation

T'ai chi chuan is another vitality-generating physical exercise. Originating in China, its aim is to allow the *chi* or vital energy to flow unhindered through the body. T'ai chi involves learning a series of precise movements that flow into each other. These stem from martial arts and are like shadow-boxing in slow motion.

Through the movements of t'ai chi you learn how to relax certain muscles rather than tense them, which helps to reduce the background tension that we all hold within our bodies. The movements also help to open up the joints, allowing the *chi* to flow unhindered. T'ai chi is therefore about developing a harmony with the self through posture and a strength through yielding. Once the sequence is learnt through attending classes with a qualified teacher, t'ai chi can be practised at home (see Resources, page 308).

You'll feel more connected and alert when you practise t'ai chi, with an inner calm. Robert, aged 66, took up t'ai chi when he retired. Here's how he describes the benefits:

> I've never been an athletic person or good at anything physical. T'ai chi, however, I enjoy immensely. I like the feeling of being 'in control' of my body. It gives me an aesthetic pleasure. I do it almost every day for 20 minutes. It increases my energy and clears my mind. It gives me a kind of equilibrium that has many benefits, such as helping me to play my violin better and helping me to stay detached when things are bad. I find it very calming when I'm stressed or feeling fraught.

Psychocalisthenics: Aerobic Yoga?

While yoga and t'ai chi are excellent natural highs, and help you maintain a level of fitness, develop some strength and stay supple, they can hardly be described as 'aerobic'. Enter *Psychocalisthenics*, the brainchild of Oscar Ichazo. Ichazo has studied and practised martial arts and yoga since 1939, as well as founding the Arica School in the 1960s as a school of knowledge for the understanding of the complete person. He thought that if you were going to spend 20 minutes a day getting fit, why not generate vital energy at the same time?

Psychocalisthenics, a routine of 23 exercises that can be done in less than 20 minutes, is a complete contemporary exercise system which, at first glance, looks like a powerful kind of aerobic yoga. 'In the same way that we have an everyday need for food and nourishment we have to promote the circulation of our vital energy as an everyday business,' says Ichazo.

So, while most exercise routines simply treat the body as a physical machine that needs to be worked to stay fit, *Psychocalisthenics* (often shortened to psychocals) is designed to generate both physical fitness and vital energy by bringing mind and body into balance. The key lies in the precise breathing pattern that accompanies each physical exercise. 'Once we integrate our mind with our body across a controlled respiration, we can produce in ourselves an element of self-observation that is indispensable for acquiring understanding of our true nature,' says Ichazo. 'What Psychocals offers is a set of exercises that can become a serious foundation for a life of self-responsibility, clarity of mind, and strength of spirit.'

The combination of movement, breath and exercises that generate vital energy is what makes Psychocals unique – a perfect combination of East and West. When we first started doing the routine (which takes a day to learn) we were amazed at how light, re-energised and 'high' we felt afterwards. Other advocates of Psychocals give the same glowing reports. 'This is exercise pared to perfection. I wasn't sweating buckets as I would after an aerobics class but I could feel I had exercised far more muscles. I was feeling clear-headed and bright rather than wiped out,' said Jane Alexander, in a *Daily Mail* review. In the USA, Psychocals is now promoted by the 'Bionic Woman', actress Lindsay Wagner.

One of the things we like most about psychocals is that you don't have to go anywhere, or wear special clothes, or buy any equipment. Once you've learnt the routine you can do it in under 20 minutes in your own home, accompanied either by the video, or with a 'talk through' music tape. It takes a day to learn and will leave you feeling blissful and energised (see Resources, page 307).

From the above it will become clear that vitality, the very real experience of feeling naturally high, is more than just the consequence of your diet, your physical fitness and state of mind. The extra factor is the one that's harder to measure, but no less tangible. Vital energy is sometimes described as the energy we draw in from the universe and, depending on how receptive we are, has the power to nourish us at a fundamental level. All the disciplines we've discussed above are designed to make us more receptive. So too is acupuncture, which works by unblocking channels of energy, called 'meridians', through which this vital energy is said to flow. When you walk by the ocean, lie on a beach, or walk in the woods on a sunny day, you feel more 'connected', more 'in touch', with a perspective on life far from the one you have, say, when commuting to work. Vital energy is that hidden ingredient that connects us with each other and with the world around us, allowing us to feel at one with it all.

Vital Energy Routine

As part of living high naturally, do one of these vital energy-generating exercises at least twice a week, if not every day:

▶ Psychocals
▶ Yoga
▶ T'ai chi

13

MEDITATION AND THE MIND

MEDITATION IS one of the best natural highs of all. It helps promote mental clarity, a sense of connection and will simultaneously increase your energy, improve your mood and keep you calm. Not only is it great for your state of mind, it also has many positive benefits for your body[1]: better responsiveness to stressful events and quicker recovery, reduced heart rate and blood pressure, a slowed rate of breathing and more stable brain-wave patterns.

Meditation has also been shown to prevent the depression of the body's immune responses that occur with stress.[2] People who practise meditation on a regular basis have been found to be less anxious, and there is little doubt that meditation and relaxation techniques are effective in dealing with anxiety, stress and insomnia.[3] This confirms research at the University of Massachusetts Medical Center that found that meditators have lower levels of the stress hormone cortisol.[4]

However, the true power of meditation in generating energy, clarity and peace goes way beyond these health benefits, gaining control over the mind, and how we respond to stress. This effect has tremendous significance because many of us are so habitually stressed that even the mildest conflicts generate an exaggerated 'fight or flight' stress reaction (see Chapter 4) more appropriately reserved for dealing with life-threatening situations. Meditation can be the way to 'unlearn' this conditioned stress response, and become less reactive to the normal stresses and strains of life.

How Meditation Balances the Brain

The starting point for meditation involves focusing your thoughts on one object, often the breath. James Thornton, director of the Heffter Research Institute, Santa Fe, New Mexico, an organisation dedicated to exploring new frontiers in neuroscience and consciousness, believes that focusing on the breath helps brings the brain into balance.[5] He explains how this works:

> Breathing is controlled by the oldest brain: the reptilian brain. The awareness [of the breath] is actually in the new brain, the neocortex. You integrate the experience of your brain by focusing the awareness in the big new human brain on the activities of the old small reptile brain and at that point, you've got a fully integrated brain functioning.

Many people experience this 'awakening' in meditation, as if everything in your life just clicks into place. The result is a whole new level of awareness and alertness – and one of the best natural highs.

But there's another part to our brains beyond the 'reptilian' and the neocortex: the middle, or mammalian, brain that connects the two. In effect this is a bridge between the higher mind and the body. Thornton believes that:

> . . . what the practice of meditation does is to allow you to integrate the experience of these three semi-autonomous brains. When they're aligned, when they're integrated, then you tend to be quite happy, then you're not pulled in different directions, and then you can open to the experience of the moment. So I think the awakened experience is actually the integrated brain functioning of these three semi-autonomous brains.

So how do you bring about this state of balance? Most meditation techniques involve focusing on one object, such as the breath or a mantra (a sound, such as 'om'). With practice, the power of the mind seems to grow and with that, your mental concentration and energy improve. This is diametrically opposed to the experience of being stressed and exhausted, in which the nature of the mind is to flit from one thing to another, leaving a trail of panic.

With regular meditation the mind becomes quieter and you become more able to focus on the task at hand, instead of dissipating your energy by trying to do many things at the same time and not really doing any of them completely. However, even this benefit is superficial compared to what happens at deeper levels of meditation.

With time and good instruction, those who meditate find they slip into an elevated state of awareness, a kind of pure 'being' in which the mind is naturally still, the body relaxed and the emotions settled. This state is real, not imagined, and correlates to a distinctive change in brain-wave patterns to a slower alpha wave rhythm. After such meditation, your energy, mental clarity and ability to stay unaffected by the turbulence of daily life are significantly greater. This is how I (Patrick) experienced one deep meditation.

I had a firsthand experience of this during a 2-day siddha yoga meditation weekend intensive. The highlight for me was on the second day when the meditation master, Gurumayi Chidvilasananda, gave a fascinating talk explaining all about the nature of the mind and how we can lose touch with the inner self. By this time, not being very good at sitting on the floor, my body was aching and my mind was tired and bursting at the seams.

Then she led us into meditation by chanting 'om'. As I did this, the sound 'om' began reverberating inside me as if my body was a vast, empty cave. The sound reverberated outside me filling the hall as if it were a magnificent cathedral. It was an extraordinary and very uplifting sensation.

Suddenly, the chanting stopped. There was not a sound. Everything went black. My mind literally stopped thinking. My body stopped aching. In fact it felt so blissful that not a single muscle stirred. There was just this delicious, empty silence. Occasionally a thought would come up like a ship on the horizon and then pass from view. I felt no emotion as such, just this pure, deep, total contentment. Every moment and every breath was so exquisite. I just sat there observing every millimetre of every breath come in, and go out, like the waves on the beach. When I opened my eyes the hall was empty and all the people had gone and I realised an hour had passed.

Since then meditation has been like dipping into a well of rejuvenating tranquillity. It has given me a place inside where I can see everything from a clearer perspective.

Oscar Ichazo, who invented *Psychocalisthenics*, is also a modern-day master of meditation. He says:

The mystical experience happens to us when and only when our cortex becomes unified or harmonised in such a way that it immediately starts working on a different level. Our mind starts going to the lowest vibrations of the EEG scale (which is a measure of the quality of brain activity). Everyone agrees that the state of meditation is produced by the alpha wave. But if we descend to the theta wave we can produce even higher states. That is when all the activities of the cerebral cortex have been pacified in a way that then it is one unity and one solid experience of our entire being. In every mystical tradition the teaching is precisely to train people to the point where they can reproduce in themselves this state of totality of the cerebral cortex.[6]

To reach this level of expertise in meditation you need to follow the instruction of a meditation master.

Instead of being blindly limited to viewing life as 'a struggle' or 'survival of the fittest', we can awaken to the oneness, the connectedness, the play of life. This is the true goal of meditation and the ultimate natural high.

Meditation Exercise

▶ Sit in a quiet place and adopt a comfortable posture with your spine straight. If you are sitting cross-legged on the floor you may find it helpful to straighten your spine by tucking a firm cushion under your pelvis.

▶ Let go of any tension in your body and feel your spine elongate.

▶ Become aware of your breath and start Dia-Kath breathing (see page 199) for nine breaths.

▶ Now let your breathing find its own rhythm. Bring your awareness to the place from where your breath arises. With each exhalation, bring your awareness to the place to where your breath goes.

▶ Whenever your mind wanders bring it back to the breath. There is no need to resist your thoughts as such – simply become aware that your focus has shifted to your thoughts and bring it back to the breath.

Remember:

▶ **Every day practise meditation for at least 10 minutes,** ideally on rising or at the end of the day. This is as refreshing as having a sleep.

▶ **Whenever you are stressed, in an unpleasant mood or feeling disconnected, practise meditation** by sitting quietly for 5 or more minutes.

If you'd like to deepen your experience of meditation, see Resources, page 305 for details of meditation courses.

14

BIOFEEDBACK, RELAXATION AND THE ALPHA STATE

Dᴵᴰ ʏᴏᴜ know that by becoming aware of your pulse rate, you can actually learn to change it? This process is called biofeedback.

For many years, scientists assumed that we were unable to voluntarily affect so-called 'autonomic' functions such as pulse rate. Then Westerners discovered yogis who could stop and start their hearts at will, and Tibetan monks who could melt huge quantities of ice with their bodies, and not appear any the worse for it. They seem to be generating endless amounts of energy, whereas if any of us tried it our bodies would become so cold we'd die. Just as these highly trained people can influence their physiology and mind states, scientists have developed powerful biofeedback technology that allows us to do similar feats.

Neurofeedback: Tame the Mind

The most direct form of biofeedback for altering your mental state is neurofeedback. It helps to tame the restless mind, promoting relaxation and balance on all levels – mental, emotional, physical and spiritual. The key is the alpha brain-wave state.

Using electrodes lightly and painlessly attached to various parts of the scalp with a special gel, the individual is hooked up to a computer-driven machine, an electroencephalograph (EEG), which detects their brain rhythms. The brain-wave patterns can then be observed on the computer screen. By seeing how changes in your internal state affect brain-wave patterns, you can learn how to shift them and train your mind to move into different states. These can range from focused attention to deep relaxation.

In a deeply relaxed, meditative state, your physical body vibrates at about 8 cycles per second (cps). At the same time, our brain waves shift from their everyday beta range (13 to 40cps) into the same 8cps deep alpha range as the body.

When this occurs, an electromagnetic field is created around the head. Amazingly, some believe this field links up with the frequency of the Earth's electromagnetic field, also hovering about 8cps. When we are in harmony with the planetary vibration, we release stress and experience a natural high!

There are many ways to get yourself into an alpha brain-wave state. You can study meditation, learn yoga, listen to specific music, or practise exercises suggested in Dr Herbert Benson's landmark book, *The Relaxation Response*. Or you can also take brain-wave biofeedback training, in which a machine monitors your body and indicates when you have achieved the necessary control of your body/mind.

One of the leading pioneers in biofeedback techniques is Dr Les Fehmi in Princeton, New Jersey. In Jim Robbins' book, *Symphony in the Brain: The Evolution of the New Brain Wave Biofeedback*, Fehmi's early research experience is described.

After weeks of frustration, going nowhere, Dr Les Fehmi once more hooked himself up to the EEG monitor. Instead of concentrating hard and focusing intently on his goal, however, this time he relaxed his focus and let go. Much to his surprise, profound feelings washed over him, and then, his life began to change dramatically. He felt far more relaxed and at ease in his body, and he adopted a more centred attitude toward life. Physical changes happened as well. Severe, long-term arthritis in his hands disappeared, and his vision and sense of smell were enhanced. He knew that this was the way life was meant to be!

Dr Fehmi continued working with himself and many others over the years, and came to the conclusion that a fundamental problem in our culture is that we are taught as children to focus too narrowly on the external world. Little support or training is given to attention-broadening pursuits. With our mind and eyes we grip objects and the outside world too intently. This leads to problems such as anxiety and depression. Fehmi now coaches people in methods to literally relax their attentional grip. As they learn to do that, the rest of the body's physiology relaxes as well.

In case you are wondering, you don't have to be wired up to an EEG monitor to benefit from Dr Fehmi's biofeedback research. He has developed a set of audio tapes that help you to move quickly into the state that produces the best brain-wave patterns. Robbins describes his own experience using these tapes.

After a couple of weeks I started noticing changes similar to those Fehmi described. A lighter feeling. More laughter. I felt more at home in my body and at times moved more fluidly. I had more energy during my noon pick-up basketball games. Some days there was an extraordinary feeling of being centred and calm, and my sense of smell was greatly enhanced. I could pick up the smell of lilacs blooming half a block away. The sun seemed more golden, richer somehow, the way I remembered it glowing from childhood. It was the first time in many years that I had felt as good. At this writing it has been about six months and the changes are still occurring as I continue to do the tapes. If I stop doing the tapes for a month or so the stress starts to build again.

Another researcher, Dr James Hardt, director of the Biocybernaut Training Institute, describes how hundreds of people have had profound spiritual experiences during the course of their Biocybernaut EEG training, with life-transforming results. He describes these in some detail on his website www.biocybernaut.com.

Another leader in the field of brain-wave training for optimal performance is Anna Wise, whose books such as *The High Performance Mind: Mastering brainwaves for insight, healing and creativity*, and CD, *The Awakened Mind*, can help you access various mind states. For details see her website www.annawise.com. There are music tapes as well: Steven Halpern's music has been shown to bring on a deep alpha state (see Resources, page 308).

Biofeedback Exercise

Find a peaceful and comfortable place to listen to an alpha wave-inducing tape or CD, such as Fehmi's *Open Focus*, Anna Wise's *Awakened Mind* or Steven Halpern's *Anti-Frantic Series*, for 20 minutes each day.

POSITIVE THINKING

MOST OF our suffering is created in our own minds. We set the scene by how we react to things that stress us out, make us feel down and zap our energy. If we feel an event is the end of world, we can become even more depressed and negative. If we look deeper, we can see that 'bad' events in life, like the end of a relationship or the loss of a job, can turn out to be blessings, both in terms of what you learn and for the space they create for new possibilities. It's this kind of positive thinking that can keep us growing, on the move and happy in our lives.

It's part of our evolutionary programming to be on the lookout for external threats. We also learn it early in life through our relationships with our parents. Think about all your negative traits. Now think about all your mother's and then all your father's negative traits. See the similarity? Early in life we learn ways of reacting to the world. These negative patterns are usually based on deep-seated false premises, such as 'No one will love me as I am', or 'I am never good enough,' or 'There is something wrong with me'. As a result, we attract situations and people that fit into our negative way of viewing life – people who abandon us or criticise us, situations in which we are destined to fail, or not live up to others' expectations. These patterns are so deep-seated that they are very hard to see. Whenever you say to yourself or others 'You never . . .' or 'You always . . .' you can be pretty certain you are seeing the situation through a deep-rooted negative pattern.

Breaking the Pattern

All this can leave us failing to express who we are, or doing the things we really want to do. We then feel bored, depressed or unfulfilled. Maybe it wasn't safe for you as a child to be angry, or you were brought up being told 'boys don't cry'. As a consequence you might say, 'I'm fine', when you're actually angry or sad.

The good news is that if we were able to learn these negative patterns, we can also unlearn them. One of the first steps to breaking the pattern is being truthful about how you feel. This can even be done in private – in your personal journal, or in an unsent letter. Releasing unexpressed emotions can liberate a lot of energy, and you then find yourself feeling lighter, even high.

You're then in a state of mind where you can replace the old negative image or belief with a positive one, such as: I am okay, I deserve to feel good, I deserve to have what I want, I am safe and protected, I can take care of myself. These are the positive messages we might have missed in childhood. But it's never too late to have a happy childhood. To the unconscious mind, time is irrelevant. You can change your inner programme, heal your inner frightened child, and live a happy life. It sounds simple, but our minds are in some ways quite basic. As you think, so you are.

Start by being good to yourself. As well as doing all the things you do for others, your partner, your friends, your children, do something for yourself. Take up a hobby or activity that you always wanted to do. Buy yourself something. Get a massage. Go for a hike. Have lunch with a friend. Go to the zoo. Do something fun, even for a short time, every day.

You can say that life isn't that kind to us, and we are always going to be faced with challenges. This is true. However, while we might not always realise it, we really can choose how we perceive and respond to difficult situations. Here's how I (Hyla) handled one such occasion.

I was driving down the Pacific Coast Highway in Malibu on my way to an appointment, with little time to spare, and traffic had come to a dead stop. I felt my jaw tighten and my breath become shallow. Trapped, I looked around for an escape route, a turn-off. My gaze was arrested by the view out my side window. The Pacific Ocean was a sparkling blue-green, the golden sand beach stretched down from the road to meet the white, crashing waves, and the bright blue sky was painted with fluffy, white clouds. 'What am I doing to myself?' I wondered.

Here, in one of the most beautiful spots I could imagine, I was complaining about being stuck in traffic! From somewhere inside me, I heard the phrase 'It's okay. I'll get there when I get there.' I put on a Steven Halpern CD. As I drank in the soothing, enlivening sound, magnificent view, and fresh saltwater smell, I could feel my jaw release and my breathing deepen. I was home, inside me – and outside, too. How could I have forgotten?

We can all do this if we just remember that we can. We can change our responses to those tough times – standing in a bank queue, cramming for a final exam or responding to a demanding 2-year-old.

And it pays to be up! Optimism and a positive attitude go a long way towards helping us maintain good health. Research shows that the higher your optimism, the healthier your immune system. Moreover, the likelier it is that good things will happen to you. Negative expectations, on the other hand, actually breed negative experiences. It sometimes takes work to be happy, not allowing yourself to give in to self-pity.

How do you incorporate these ideas and practices into your own life? You can begin by being grateful. You know the saying 'count your blessings'? Well, do it – literally. We all have a lot to be grateful for. And no matter how bad things might appear, there is always someone who has worse problems. In fact, reaching out to such people will most likely help you at least as much as it helps them.

You can also do it yourself. See the following box for specific exercises.

Positive Programming

▶ **Resolve an issue** you have with someone. Write a comprehensive letter expressing all your negative feelings about them, going through every emotionally charged incident with them, really letting rip, holding nothing back, telling them that you won't accept their behaviour. Don't send it. Now write a letter detailing everything you like about them, how much you've learned from them, going through every incident you can recall where you felt uplifted and supported by them. Don't send it. This simple exercise will make you clearer and more able to meet them and resolve the issue. In fact, when you're done with it, you may have lost the entire emotional charge, and can just laugh it off.

▶ **Say how you feel.** When someone asks you how you are, say how you *really* feel, not just the usual 'good, fine, great'. When you have an emotional charge with someone, you can tell them that, 'When you said or did X, I felt Y, and I would prefer that you do or say Z.' If you're pissed off about something, beat up a pillow, go kick-boxing, scream your head off or whatever you need to do to get it out of your system.

▶ **Create your own reality.** Visualise what you want to happen, while in a state of deep relaxation. This actually draws the experience to you by keeping you focused on your ideal goal.

We are fortunate to have many resources that can help in the process, as well. You can work, one to one, with a psychotherapist, or take courses specifically designed to help you work through and move beyond self-limiting negative patterns, or you can read books on the subject. In the Recommended Reading section on page 303 we list our favourites, based both on our own experience and the feedback of others. There is something for everyone. For Resources, see page 306.

16

THE POWER OF TOUCH

WITHOUT TOUCH, we die. Really. Years ago, psychologists observing babies in orphanages noted that, though fed and given rudimentary care, many of them simply wasted away and died. The missing ingredient here was touch. Staffing was very limited, and no one had time for the holding and cuddling that these babies needed to sustain their young lives. Those who did manage to survive were emotionally and physically stunted for life. Other classic research isolated baby monkeys in cages with two 'mothers': a wire one with a rubber nipple that fed them milk, and a terry-cloth one that did not feed them. When frightened, these little monkeys clung to the cloth surrogate. So cuddles are as vital as food.

Of course the vast majority of us know how wonderful it feels to be held in someone's arms: we don't need scientific reports to know that touch nurtures our bodies and souls. By raising our endorphin levels, it can lift us into bliss. Any mother calming a frightened child could tell us this.

It's not just hugs and caresses that can help us here. Massage has been an integral part of healing practices the world over for centuries. Western medicine has lost the art, though it is gaining increasing recognition these days. In fact, researchers at Miami, Duke and Harvard Universities and at Miami's Touch Research Institute have done numerous controlled studies showing that massage has remarkable benefits in treating a whole host of conditions. For example, premature infants massaged three times a day for 10 days gained weight 47 per cent faster than a control group. Although their consumption of formula milk was equal, the massaged babies appeared better able to absorb and utilise it.

At Columbia Presbyterian Hospital, New York, under the leadership of the innovative heart specialist Dr Mehmet Oz, massage is being used regularly on patients who've had open heart surgery and heart transplants. Results show that healing time and complications are greatly reduced. For details, read Oz's fascinating book, *Healing from the Heart*. In it, Oz reports a case where he was able to resuscitate the failing heart of a young patient just out of cardiac surgery. Unresponsive to the usual efforts, the patient rallied when the doctor massaged his feet vigorously for 45 minutes. This is fascinating, as it upholds a major finding of reflexology – that acupressure points related to all parts of the body cluster thickly on the soles of the feet. Oz was helping the patients' heart along by stimulating the right point on his feet![1]

Try this simple exercise: Hold your partner's hand in both of yours, and just feel – the warmth, contours, subtle pulsation of blood flow. After a few minutes, let go and ask how his or her hand feels, compared to the other one. Invariably, the touched hand feels more vibrant, alive, energised, as if it has been massaged. And you accomplished that with no movement at all.

The Magic of Massage

My (Hyla's) friend Jane recounted the following adventure that illustrates the magic of receiving and connecting through massage.

I had an amazing massage experience at the Esalen Institute in Big Sur, California. It was January in the late 1980s. There was blue sky above, green mountains in the background and the azure ocean below, stretching as far as the eye could see. I was already feeling pretty good (and who wouldn't, in this place?) when I entered the massage room. In the background was music that almost instantly calmed my mind and nurtured my spirit. The therapist introduced himself, and I knew from the first touch that this was going to be special. I could feel the energy flow from his hand, and back from my body in response, and so it continued – a positive feedback loop of bliss! My breathing and heart rate slowed down, the tight muscles in my body surrendered, and my mind was silenced, far from its usual preoccupations. Time disappeared, as we did a silent, intimate tango over the next hour. This delicious dance came to a gentle end – too soon, of course. When we said good-bye, he confided to me that, after four years, this was his last massage there. He was leaving that day, and he had really put his heart and soul into this special occasion.

The very special and intimate nature of such massage begs the question: was there a sexual overtone, especially with this being a man giving a massage to a woman? This is an issue that comes up for those who haven't had much experience with massage. The answer is that the experience did have a sensual aspect to it. When asked the question, Jane responded that, in fact, she felt alive and all in contact with her masseur through all her body. And beyond that, with the cosmos.

Coming back to Earth, though, let's address the issue of sex versus the sensual. Children and animals are uninhibited in experiencing their sensuality. Cats stretch, love to be stroked and kids will tickle each other and giggle for hours. Sensuality is a natural expression of who we are, and need not lead to sex.

In choosing a massage partner, or even in sharing a hug, be aware that the issue may arise, and be sure that clear boundaries and intentions are in place before you begin. In our culture, because touch is not an integral part of life (as it is in much of the rest of the world), we may confuse it with sexuality. Sex may be the only time many people do have physical contact. This leaves out the many people who are without partners, without sexual opportunities, or even, without a desire for sex. But they may well want to be touched and hugged.

A friend of mine, a radio show host, told me about an experience he had with his 98-year-old grandmother:

A couple of years ago, I was visiting my grandmother. She was still sharp, but severely limited by her hearing, sight and mobility. As we talked quietly – as quietly as you can talk to the near-deaf – I gently rubbed her back. She became nearly tearful, as she thanked me and told me how good that felt. I don't recall if she said directly that she didn't get touched enough, but it was clear to me.

The two things that stick with me are, first, the bond created between us in the way her body being touched, touched her heart. I felt it awoke something from years before, perhaps even from her youth. And, secondly, I realised that this moment is waiting to happen for millions of seniors, millions of our mothers and fathers.

The healing power of touch knows no age limits.

Give, Receive or Keep It All for Yourself

Learning how to massage is like learning to play a musical instrument. Once you master the basic notes and chords, you can then improvise, and let the music come from within. Your movements are the technique, the body you massage the instrument, and it's the interaction between the two that makes the music. The communication is intimate, almost sacred, as your two consciousnesses connect. As one giving a massage, be sensitive, tune in to your partner. And don't assume you have to know anything, or be an expert. Even professionals will check in repeatedly, both verbally and more subtly by watching body language. Otherwise, ask the person for feedback.

If both giver and receiver synchronise their breathing rhythms, massage can be more effective. It's as if you actually share the same breath, and this increases rapport and receptivity. Steven Halpern reports that massage professionals notice that they don't feel as tired at the end of a long day when they play his music. In fact, a recent article acknowledged that, of the top 25 albums for massage, his recordings 'were in a class by themselves – and highly recommended'. (We recommend you try Halpern's *Comfort Zone, Music For Sound Healing* or *Spectrum Suite*; see Resources, page 308.)

When you're receiving a massage, the first moment of physical contact tells you a lot about what's to come. When the massage therapist is closely attuned to you and your body, this moment can be almost sacred. It is a shared meeting with another human being, which just doesn't happen often enough in our fast and stressful modern world.

Take advantage of this initial contact by tuning in especially closely to what's happening in your own body. You also pick up information about the person who is touching you. Focus on your breathing and on relaxing.

As each new part is touched breathe into it, picturing the tension melting away, releasing more and more deeply with each breath. Communicate about what feels good and not – 'that feels good, and could you do it a little more lightly?' or 'a little stronger or lower, higher . . .'. You get the picture. Really allow yourself to receive, without guilt. (See Resources, page 305, for access to good massage therapists.)

But what if you live alone and don't have access to a massage partner or therapist? Self massage is an excellent option. A great book on this is Jaqueline Young's *Self Massage*. Try massaging your own hands and feet, for example. Put on some music, light candles, use some aromatic oils and you are off and running (or actually, the opposite). You would be surprised at how relaxing, even blissful this can be. Another option: trade massages with a friend or relative.

Massage Exercise

Book yourself a massage or do it yourself by creating your own special 'Massage Temple' setting. These are the suggested ingredients:

▶ A quiet, private, comfortable room.

▶ A massage table, floor or table appropriately padded, or simply a bed, if with an intimate partner – or otherwise, if you have set the appropriate boundaries.

▶ Massage oil – apricot, almond or another natural product. Never use petroleum-based products. They are unhealthy.

▶ Music (see the list on pages 246–7).

▶ Candles.

▶ Incense or essential oils (see page 239).

Not much time? Exchange foot rubs with a friend. Or back rubs. It does not have to be a full-on, total body, hourly thing every time.

Remember to connect as either giver or receiver. The experience is there for the giving and the taking. We have a huge capacity to give and receive. The secret is the awareness of this potential gift, the willingness to surrender, and the belief that we deserve to feel this good!

17

SEXUAL CHEMISTRY

ONE OF the most pleasurable highs we have is sex, in all its many forms and flavours. It can be soft, warm, and cuddly; wild and passionate; or divinely spiritual. It can be all of these at once. We will have a look at the full array of sensuality and sexuality, fantasy, lust, love, tenderness and passion. While we won't pretend we have all the answers to this great mystery called sex, we can describe its range, its effects, ways to enjoy and enhance it, and its accompanying brain and body chemistry. (Only if it matters to you. Otherwise, you can skip that section and go straight to the action part.)

Sex is as complex as we are, shifting with our moods, our age, the perfume of that amazing-looking young waitress, or the smile of a man who just strolled by. A 'certain look' from your lover from across the room might get you more turned on than by full-on sexual contact. What is this mystery called sex?

Human beings do not mate only to procreate: sex permeates every aspect of our lives. Most animals have sex only for reproduction, with some exceptions. Dolphins, for example, display a range of sensuality and sexuality in their playful interactions, and will even include unsuspecting human beings who are innocently swimming near them. Women have reported being pursued relentlessly by a male dolphin who rubbed himself unashamedly against their skin, and appeared to want more.

The Chemistry of Sex: Hormone Heaven

First we will look at the hormones and neurotransmitters that orchestrate the complex sexual dance, in all its shadings. Here is a look at the major players.

DHEA (page 43) is an anti-ageing, energising, anti-stress hormone that can also convert to both oestrogen and testosterone. Not only does it stimulate the sexual response, it even stimulates the production of pheromones. As we reveal in the aromatherapy chapter, these are special chemicals that our skin secretes in order to attract the opposite sex via their sense of smell.[1] We can enhance their effect by wearing them in combination with certain essential oils, such as ylang ylang, vanilla and musk.

Meanwhile, the pituitary gland in the brain puts out oxytocin, prolactin and vasopressin, each with its own role in this drama. The 'bonding hormone' oxytocin makes a couple want to touch and cuddle, and contributes to monogamy. In women, it leads to the contractions of orgasm, and in men, it speeds ejaculation and promotes a post-orgasmic relaxation response, followed all too rapidly by sleep. Prolactin, also released during breast-feeding, increases during orgasm, then dips. Vasopressin, especially in men, helps to maintain mental focus, read sexual clues, and avoid extreme behaviours, such as getting distracted by another woman in mid-flirtation. (That probably happens anyway, vasopressin notwithstanding.)

The feel-good neurotransmitter phenethylamine (PEA), also found in chocolate (page 79), is the 'love chemical'. It helps to create a feeling of excitement and turn-on. In men, visual cues will set it off, and lust is born. Then along comes the motivator, dopamine, urging the man to ask for her phone number. His fantasies about her raise his level of male sex hormone, testosterone, among other things, as this hormone cocktail shunts his rational mind due south. Testosterone also drives female libido. (Decreasing levels as women approach the menopause are a major factor behind decreased sexual desire.) During and especially just after orgasm, the endorphins kick in, and ecstatic feelings prevail.

We have just caught a glimpse of the complex chemical orchestra that makes all kinds of music, changing volume, beat and harmony, as the various hormonal instruments move into and out of prominence. How can we best preserve and enjoy this symphony and use it for our elevation? Of course, the flipside occurs. We can use and degrade or downgrade sex, like alcohol, to dissipate energy and avoid pain.

Good sex, however, is high on the list of natural highs, both as a relaxant and as a means to connection. The more you are in the moment, tuning in to all your senses and sensations, the better the experience. This harks back to ancient cultures, where sacred sexuality was honoured, as opposed to Western society's artificial schism between sex and spirit. The split has led only to guilt for having these normal inclinations, and repression of desire.

In practising sacred sexuality, on the other hand, we have an opportunity to reconnect with ourselves and our partner in a deep and powerful way. This not only renews and re-energises us, but brings us closer to the essence of who we are. This practice can enhance creativity, love, knowledge, empowerment, passion and a celebration of life. To quote Margo Anand, author of *The Art of Sexual Ecstasy*, 'Ecstasy transcends sex. Every moment is pregnant with ecstasy'.

Don't Forget to Play

Sex is one area where we can also be playful, silly, creative and spontaneous. Despite all the serious aspects that we just discussed, don't forget to just have a good time – on your own, or with a partner.

Sex can't exactly be orchestrated. As in learning to dance, the right moves will become second nature, and you will discover all kinds of creative things to do. There are also many tapes and books that give you a series of exercises that build on each other, to help expand your range of sexual feelings and repertoire of activities. Here are some guidelines for creating a conducive atmosphere. Your own preferences will, of course, work the best.

Sex Exercises

1. Sex is not limited to physical sexual contact, or to the bedroom. Set the stage as far in advance as you can stand.

2. Leave a love-note for your partner, inviting them to a mysterious evening encounter. Send him or her flowers during the day. Leave a provocative message on their answering machine.

3. Have a candle-lit dinner, romantic music in the background, finger food that you feed lovingly to each other (don't stop to do the dishes) . . . a bubble bath filled with essential oils, aphrodisiacs such as vanilla, musk or ylang ylang.

4. Maintain eye contact as much as you can (without tripping on the stairs), and feel the charge building up between you.

5. By the time you get to the bedroom, you will have been engaged in sex for hours! Try a slow massage – hands, feet, back, neck. You might want to change the music at some point, too, to something more rhythmic.

6. You get the picture. Sex is not just sex!

LIGHT AND COLOUR

EVER WONDERED why a holiday in the sun leaves you feeling so high? It may all have been down to the positive effects of natural sunlight. Many people suffer from light deficiency. Some are more susceptible than others, and consequently are more prone to low moods, especially in the winter. There is now plenty of evidence that increasing light exposure boosts your mental performance as well as your mood.[1]

One of the pioneers of light therapy was the late Francis Lefebure, who developed a technique known as phosphenism.[2] Phosphenes are the after-images that are seen when you close your eyes after looking at a light source. He studied this phenomenon and was able to demonstrate that various exercises that involved closing your eyes and focusing on these after-images could stimulating learning, mood, motivation and creativity. Unfortunately, his work has not been followed up, despite impressive results. We include one very simple phosphenic exercise at the end of this chapter that can be very helpful for those prone to low moods, especially in the winter.

Light also boosts your immune system. This is because it stimulates skin cells to produce a very powerful immune-boosting substance, interleukin-1 (IL-1).[3] IL-1 is stimulated by natural daylight, which is a good reason to spend some time every day outdoors exposing yourself, so to speak.

What is it about natural sunlight that makes it different from indoor lighting? Natural sunlight is a full spectrum of different wavelengths that create a 'white' light. Rainbows show the different wavelengths broken up as bands of colour which collectively make what we perceive as white light. Light bulbs are not the same thing. They contain a narrower band of wavelengths, and the light is more 'yellow' as a result. Fluorescent lighting is closer. The best indoor lighting, however, is called 'full-spectrum' lighting, and it aims to mimic the wavelengths of natural light, and its benefits. If you work indoors with little exposure to natural light, it's worth investing in full-spectrum lighting. (See Resources, page 305, for suppliers.)

A Healthy Colour

Colours influence your mood. Research in schools investigating the effects of changing the colours in classrooms has shown that yellow, orange and red increase IQ and stimulate learning, while black and brown have the opposite effect and green is neutral.[4] Blue, on the other hand, has been shown to calm down hyperactive children.[5] The effects of exposing yourself to different hues of light is likely to be even more powerful. Colour is used in a variety of ways for healing and the general consensus is that the following colours tend to have the following effects, although colour therapists stress that people do respond differently to each colour.

Violet	Connects. Peaceful. Meditative. Helps balance the mind.
Magenta	Connects. Energising. Self-empowering.
Blue	Relaxes. Calms body and mind. Antidote to stress.
Turquoise	Relaxes. Soothing. Refreshing. Eases anxiety.
Orange	Stimulates. Cheerful, mood enhancing. More relaxing.
Red	Stimulates. Invigorating, activating. More exhausting.
White	Stimulator, mood booster, mind enhancer and connector.

You can put this information to good use by having 'soft' lights for your evening lighting emitting turquoise, blue, magenta or violet colour ranges.

Candlelight, which is of a much lower intensity, is also much more calming than strong daylight. For your 'day' lighting, make sure you have plenty of it, either as good natural daylight or full-spectrum light bulbs.

Light Exercise

This exercise is particularly effective for those prone to depression, especially during the winter, when there is less natural daylight.

▶ Sit down in a quiet place, on the floor or on a chair. It is best to choose a place that you can completely darken. If not, you will need a blindfold.

▶ Place an angle-poise lamp, containing a 60 watt opaque (not clear) bulb, preferably with no writing on it, 3 feet away and directly in front of your line of vision.

▶ Make sure you can turn the light on and off without moving your head position.

▶ Turn the light on and look directly at the bulb for 1 minute, no longer.

▶ After 1 minute, turn the light off, close your eyes (put on your blindfold if the room is not completely dark) and focus on the after-image, the phosphene, without moving your head, until it completely vanishes. This usually takes 3 to 4 minutes.

19

AROMATHERAPY

SMELL EVOKES emotion and memory like no other sense. One sniff of a childhood constant – freshly baked bread, tomato soup, a certain kind of flower your mother grew, a particular kind of soap – can conjure up images of the past, even whole chapters of our lives. And we're drawn especially to certain smells that remind us of happy times – the cinnamon and cloves of hot punch at Christmas, the scent of pinewoods or the salt tang of the sea. So smell is a very special key that can be used to open certain doors in the mind.

The term 'aromatherapy' was first coined in the early part of the twentieth century by the French chemist René-Maurice Gattefossé to describe the medicinal use of essential oils. These oils are the vital essence or 'soul' of the plant, containing their concentrated therapeutic and nutritional compounds, including phytohormones. Just as in humans, these are chemical messengers that act throughout the plant in response to environmental conditions, including stress. These plant hormones can affect us, too, when we inhale their fragrance, apply them topically or orally ingest them. In fact, many traditional herbal remedies had multiple purposes – a single potion often served as perfume, a topical salve and an oral medicine.

Scientific evidence supporting aromatherapy is just beginning to surface. In a 1992 issue of the *British Journal of Occupational Therapy*, aromatherapy is described as a treatment to 'promote health and well-being' through massage, inhalation, baths and the application of compresses, creams and lotions. This suggests that fragrance can reduce stress and depression, sedate or invigorate, stimulate sensory awareness and provide pain relief. Researchers have found that fragrance can even improve interaction and communication among people: pleasant smells can put people in better moods and make them more willing to negotiate, cooperate and compromise than they would be in a scent-free room.

The Knowing Nose

How does smell affect us so deeply and immediately? Smell is the most basic of senses. In the animal world it means survival – searching for food, sniffing danger or finding a mate. While we may not be aware of using our olfactory sense in this way, it does, in fact, have a powerful effect on us. Smells are carried directly by the olfactory nerves to the limbic system, a primitive part of the brain that acts as a kind of emotional switchboard. The limbic system evaluates sensory stimuli, and registers pleasure or pain, safety or danger, with corresponding emotional responses such as anger, fear, repulsion or attraction. This response then connects to the part of the brain that influences memory, learning, basic emotions, hormonal balances and even our basic survival mechanisms, such as the 'fight or flight' response.

In the brain a particular scent unlocks and retrieves specific memories associated with it, often many years old, since the sense of smell has the longest recall of all the senses. So as we've said, scents can be a direct pathway to memory and emotion. Fragrances can relieve pain, call up deep-seated memories and generally affect personality and behaviour.

Using oil fragrances may turn out to be one of the fastest ways to achieve psychological results, too. 'Smells act directly on the brain, like a drug,' says Dr Alan Hirsch, a neurologist, psychiatrist and director of the Smell and Taste Treatment and Research Center in Chicago. Scientific research supports the notion that smelling particular odours has a direct effect on brain activity.

Oil on Troubled Waters

We can see how different scents produce specific emotional states, communicated through the various neurotransmitters. Marjoram, for example, is a sedating oil, stimulating the secretion of the calming transmitter serotonin. Dr J. J. King, a psychiatrist at the Smallwood Day Hospital in Redditch, Worcestershire, has successfully treated anxiety with aromatherapy. He uses pleasant, natural scents that are known relaxants such as lavender, rose, bergamot, cypress and balsam fir, and combines them with relaxation techniques such as deep breathing, positive visualisation, soothing music and heat treatments. Once patients learn to associate a particular fragrance with deep relaxation, they relax whenever they are given a sniff. So, in addition to the intrinsic qualities of the oils themselves, he has added a 'conditioned response'. That is, the body and mind are trained through association of the smell with the relaxed state.

One way to measure this is to monitor certain brain waves with an electroencephalograph, or EEG. 'We know from brain-wave frequency studies that smelling lavender increases alpha waves in the back of the head, which are associated with relaxation,' says Dr Hirsch. Research has also found that brain waves slow down when you smell certain fragrances. The scents that proved to have the greatest sedative effect were (in order of effectiveness): lavender, bergamot, marjoram, sandalwood, lemon and chamomile. Scientists at the Japanese fragrance firm Takasago also measured brain waves to determine levels of relaxation produced by lavender.

According to research by Dr Susan Schiffman, professor of medical psychology at Duke University in North Carolina, sedative drugs such as Valium and Librium affect a newly discovered group of smell receptors in the brain. She reasons that if smell receptors help to sedate us, the fragrance itself should perform similarly. To test her theory, she sprayed spicy scents into New York City subway cars to see if that relaxed the passengers enough to improve their dispositions. After comparing the number of pushes, shoves and nasty comments in scented cars to those in unscented cars, she found that certain fragrances appeared to cut aggressive acts almost in half. Sounds like an excellent idea!

Refreshing Mood-boosters

Sixteenth- and seventeenth-century herbalists in Europe used clary sage and lemon balm to counter mental fatigue and depression, and they are still used for this purpose today. These simple drug-free anti-depressants may eventually be accepted by medical doctors as well. According to recent research by biochemist George Dodd and psychologist Steve van Toller at the Warwick Olfaction Research Group in England, the effect of fragrance on the brain is similar to that of some antidepressant drugs. This means that certain scents, such as orange, alter the brain chemistry behind depression, anxiety and probably other mood changes.

Aromatic Uppers

People whose jobs depend on their staying alert, such as long-distance truck drivers, can now sniff specific formulas to help them do so. Train conductors in Japan and Russia use an 'odorphone' developed by Russian professor of biology and odorologist, V. Krasnov. The little machine spews out hot whiffs of pine, cedar, rose or even seaweed or mushroom, as required. Air New Zealand and Virgin Atlantic airlines have even developed kits of floral-scented bath oils to reduce jet lag, available to passengers at London's Heathrow Airport.

Some of the first investigations into fragrant stimulants were done in the 1920s by Italian psychiatrists Giovanni Gatti and Renato Cayola. They found that the scents of clove, ylang-ylang, cinnamon, lemon, cardamom, fennel and angelica were stimulating. Peppermint and eucalyptus can also be stimulating. Later, when brain waves were recorded by researcher Shizuo Torii of the Toho University School of Medicine in Tokyo, they showed that some of these fragrances and numerous others – basil, jasmine, black pepper and, to a lesser degree, rose, patchouli, lemongrass and sage – also acted as stimulants. They tend to increase beta waves in the front of the head, which are associated with a more alert state.

These healthy stimulants not only don't trigger the stress response, but also actually counter the typical adrenal response caused by caffeine, stress and other common stimulative triggers. They also relieve drowsiness, irritability and headaches. Dr Torii has found that by arousing the autonomic nervous system, which controls breathing and blood pressure, stimulating fragrances help to maintain your attention, which generally lags after 30 minutes of sustained concentration.

To test the effects of such fragrances on alertness, researchers William Dember and Joel Warm gave people at the University of Cincinnati a stressful 40-minute task based on identifying patterns on a computer. Those working in rooms scented with peppermint had many more correct answers than people working in unscented rooms. In addition, their performance levels didn't decline as rapidly. In a study conducted by researchers at Rensselaer Polytechnic Institute in Troy, New York, clerical workers set specific goals for themselves and were more efficient when their offices were specifically scented. The fragrance worked even when those taking the test did not think that the scent was influencing them.

Scent and Sex

Aphrodisiac scents such as jasmine and ylang ylang stimulate the pituitary gland to secrete endorphins, which relay feelings of relaxation, bliss and expanded consciousness to our brains.

Some fragrances – including ylang ylang, rose, patchouli, sandalwood, jasmine, vanilla and musk – are both relaxing and stimulating. Although it might seem as if these effects would cancel each other out, they actually combine to produce a very enjoyable mood. Since stress and tension are strong deterrents to passion, the state of being completely relaxed yet stimulated offers the perfect combination for an aphrodisiac. Other aphrodisiacs include the stimulants cinnamon and coriander – used for this purpose in *The Arabian Nights*.

The association of scent and sex comes as no surprise. All animals, humans included, utilise the sex-scent 'pheromone' molecules to attract or find a potential mate. Produced in specialised apocrine or sweat glands, they are picked up by the minute vomeronasal organ in the nose. The signal is then transmitted to the limbic system, creating a sexual response. Researchers have exposed people in public places and offices to pheromone extracts. The results are a noticeable increase in friendly behaviour. In one experiment, a pair of identical twin women was sent to a singles bar, with only one wearing a pheromone extract. Video cameras capturing the action showed that the scented twin had far more men make overtures, while by comparison, her equally attractive sister was practically a wallflower. And, as in nature, these men had no idea what had hit them.

Transcendent Scents

Life energy – variously known as *chi* in China, bioplasma in Russia or vital force in the parlance of homeopathy – is the metaphysical aspect of our body. It is said that essential oils promote strengthening of this invisible energy field, the aura, in which we exist, and through which we all connect. When combined with the healing touch of massage, it will literally expand the aura, as seen on Kirlian photographs, a method of measuring electrical energy by its image on film. Mystics and spiritual teachers have always known this, and many religious traditions have included the use of essential oils in their rituals.

Essential Oils: The Essentials

Essential oils are ideal for skin care, massage, and mental and emotional rejuvenation. But some people, especially those allergic to perfumes, may be sensitive to certain essences. You can safely 'patch-test' essential oils by placing a couple of drops on the back of your hand.

It's vital to buy good-quality natural essential oils. True essential oils emit full, complex fragrances that are nearly impossible to duplicate in the laboratory. No synthetic copy, regardless of its derivation, can match the precise blend of chemicals found in an essential oil. Even slight changes will unbalance the fragrance, and, by upsetting delicate synergies, eliminate or reduce their therapeutic value. The only way to be sure of the quality of a fragrance is to purchase from a reputable supplier.

You need to blend pure essential oils with a 'carrier' oil (refined, expeller-pressed vegetable oils such as almond oil), adding 5ml (0.2 fl oz) of essence to 115ml (4 fl oz) of carrier oil, to produce aromatic oil for massage or perfume. For bath oils it is better to use half as much carrier oil, blending 5ml of essence with 60ml (2 fl oz) of carrier oil.

Here are some useful suggestions for blends.

▶ **Massage**: Used for relaxation (lavender, orange, marjoram, chamomile) or to ease muscular pain (chamomile, lavender). Select your carrier oil according to skin type: oily (apricot, walnut, soy), dry (olive, almond, cocoa butter), normal (corn, sesame, sunflower).

▶ **Bath**: Add 7 to 8 drops of a soothing essence (chamomile, rose, orange, lavender, sandalwood, ylang ylang) to a hot bath, to waft your troubles away.

▶ **Room scenting**: You can enjoy the psychological benefits of essential oils while refreshing and purifying indoor air by diffusing essences with aroma lamps or electric diffusers. Aroma lamps warm essential oils in water over a candle, evaporating their scent into the air. Diffusers emit atomised essential oil and small amounts of deodorising ozone.

▶ **Perfume**: Before synthetics, perfumes were made by blending essential oils with vegetable oils and animal scents such as musk. Make your own by adding a few drops of essence to carrier oil. For attracting the opposite sex, use a pheromone-spiked formula (but be prepared for the consequences).

Overleaf are some formulas you can make yourself, or see Resources on page 305 for supplies and sources of information.

Aromatherapy Exercise

Depending on what you need, use one of the following formulas in your bath, for scenting your room, as perfume or for massage.

Relaxant Fragrance

115ml (4 fl oz) sweet almond oil
10 drops each lavender and lemon essential oils
2 drops each marjoram and sandalwood essential oils

Mood-booster Fragrance

115ml (4 fl oz) sweet almond oil
10 drops each bergamot and petitgrain essential oils
3 drops rose geranium essential oil
1 drop neroli essential oil (expensive, so it's optional)

Stimulant for Fatigue

115ml (4 fl oz) sweet almond oil
15 drops lemon essential oil
4 drops eucalyptus essential oil
1 drop each cinnamon, peppermint, clove, patchouli, benzoin or sage essential oils (as available)

Memory Stimulant

115ml (4 fl oz) sweet almond oil
10 drops each lavender and lemon essential oils
5 drops rosemary essential oil
1 drop cinnamon essential oil

Aphrodisiac

115ml (4 fl oz) sweet almond oil
10 drops each lavender and sandalwood essential oils
2 drops each ylang ylang and vanilla essential oils
1 drop each cinnamon and jasmine essential oils

Lavender is not an aphrodisiac, but is added to make the fragrance more mellow. It can be a relaxing and emotionally uplifting scent. If you love the fragrance of patchouli, you can · use it in place of ylang ylang.

Connecting Scents

A combination of relaxing and aphrodisiac scents will do the trick. Here is where you can experiment with your own recipes . . .

20

THE MUSIC OF
THE EMOTIONS

'Music has charms to soothe a savage breast.'

William Congreve (1670–1729)

'... Half an hour of music produces the same effect as ten milligrams of Valium.'

Raymond Bahr, Director of Coronary Care,
St Agnes Hospital, Baltimore, Maryland

You know how a special song can transport you back in time to a very specific experience, one that you can actually feel in your body? Think of a hit song from your teenage years, when you were beginning to experience so many new aspects of the world. Does it get your emotions – or your hormones – flowing? Does your heart break all over again when they play a song that you listened to when you split from a partner? On a more up note, do you feel your heart opening wide when you hear the strains of 'Ode to Joy' from Beethoven's Ninth Symphony?

Sound is a powerful key to our bodies and psyches. Although its role in the West is largely entertainment, for thousands of years people throughout the world have used music to heal the body, mind and spirit. Only recently has the field of 'sound healing' emerged once again into public awareness. Recent studies have shown that music can reduce stress, enhance immune system function, slow down and balance brain-wave activity, reduce muscle tension, increase endorphin levels, and evoke feelings of love and inner peace. Pretty good for something as available as your nearest CD player or radio!

We've Got Rhythm

Although there are many paths to healing, the common denominator in most approaches is that the body heals itself most effectively in a state of deep relaxation. Specific relaxation techniques are usually necessary, as opposed to simply 'doing nothing', or watching TV. People may *think* they are achieving meaningful relaxation, but they are often mistaken. One of the simplest and most effective ways to evoke 'the relaxation response', a term coined by Dr Herbert Benson in his landmark book of the same name, is through the use of music. The most powerful effect of music is our physical response to 'the beat'. The phenomenon known as 'rhythm entertainment' describes how an external rhythmic stimulus, such as a ticking clock, drum or pulse in a musical composition, involuntarily causes your heartbeat to match its speed.

Innovative new-age composer Steven Halpern has been a leader and researcher in the field of sound and healing since 1970. He writes that:

> At age 22, I was already a classic Type A individual. Given my background as an ex-New Yorker, it was not surprising that my requirement was 'I want my relaxation – and I want it now!' I needed a solution – something legal, non-addictive and effective, available at my convenience and virtually instantaneous. (Does this sound familiar?) The solution was to combine my training in music and psychology with insights ranging from ancient shamanic sound traditions to modern bio-physics and vibrational medicine.

We now have an extensive body of research that has measured and validated the psychological and physiological benefits of music on human development and behaviour. For example, as we've seen, in a state of deep relaxation or meditation, the electromagnetic field surrounding our head literally entrains and attunes to the basic electromagnetic field of the Earth itself! The Earth's harmonic resonance has been measured at approximately 8 cycles per second, or 8 hertz (Hz). The frequency range of the electrical activity of the brain that we access in states of deep relaxation is also centred around 8Hz. This is why we feel so rejuvenated when surrounded by nature in a forest, in the mountains, or by the ocean.

Music has the power to restore our connection with our essence and with the cosmos. According to Halpern, who was among the first to use sound and music to shift brain waves into alpha and theta states to induce relaxation, 'Being in harmony with oneself and the Universe may be more than a poetic concept.' It is in the stillness that we align and attune to the deeper spiritual dimensions of life. It is in the stillness that true healing occurs. There is no need to 'do' anything; all you need is to 'be' with the music. Halpern's music and others are listed on pages 246–7.

Chemistry of Sound

At the Addiction Research Center in Stanford, California, people listened to various kinds of music, including marching bands, spiritual anthems and movie soundtracks. About half the listeners reported feelings of euphoria, leading the researchers to suspect that the joy of music is linked to the release of endorphins. To test this theory, investigators injected listeners with naloxone, which blocks opiate (endorphin) receptors. Sure enough, the listeners experienced far less pleasure. This suggests that certain types of music can actually boost endorphins.[1]

There is also research on the effects of music on stress levels. Clinical psychologist and music therapist Mark Rider tested corticosteroid levels of 12 shift-working nurses under high stress. As you may recall, these hormones are secreted by our adrenal glands during the fight-or-flight stress response. He also took body temperatures to assess the degree to which their bodies retained proper circadian (day/night) rhythms – an indicator of body-mind homeostasis or inner balance. When the nurses listened to tapes of soothing music and practised relaxation and guided imagery, their rhythms were appropriately balanced and their levels of stress hormones were reduced. On days when the nurses did not listen to the tapes, their rhythms were out of balance and their stress hormones were significantly higher.

This is reflected in the words of Dr Mitchell Gaynor in *Sounds of Healing*:

> I am convinced that each of us has our own perfect, inborn biofeedback monitor that tells us what sounds will have the most salutary influence on our cardiovascular, immune and nervous systems, not to mention our emotional and spiritual selves.

Ecstasy Through Music

Relaxation is not the only state that music can induce. When we can't stop moving to an insistent samba beat, or leap up from our seats at a rock concert, we are also responding to the power of music to literally move us. From chanting dervishes who whirl their way into ecstatic dance to young clubbers, we are all doing what comes naturally. Feeling down? Put on an upbeat CD, and let the beat take over. Here is a quote from Joel S., a 45-year-old successful business activist (someone who espouses socially aware business practices) and sometime drummer:

> I find drumming a deep cleansing, a harmonisation, and alignment of my cellular structure with the rhythm and groove. If people are dancing, I need to consciously relax myself, breathe, and allow the energy to go through me – or I will explode. Then, I end up smiling uncontrollably – both while I'm drumming and for some time afterwards. I'm high!

You can use music consciously to alter your state – as a natural stimulant, relaxant, mood booster and connector, both at home and at work. Relaxation and work are not contradictory concepts. Many people spend 45 per cent or more of their waking state in their offices, and the demand for efficiency and effectiveness continues to grow. Using the right musical background can actually promote your productivity and creativity, while simultaneously maintaining your energy and uplifting your sense of overall well-being.

Music Exercise

Here are some suggestions of music to relax, stimulate or uplift, enhancing your mood and sense of connection. Our all-time favourites are in **bold**. (R = relaxing; S = stimulating; U = uplifting)

MAINLY INSTRUMENTAL

R/U	**Siddha Yoga**	**Remembrance**	*www.siddhayoga.org*
R/U	**Peter Gabriel**	**Passion**	*Uni/Geffen*
U	**Mark Knopfler**	**Screenplaying**	*Warner Brothers*
R	Paul Horn	Inside Taj Mahal	*Kuckuck Records*
R/U	Gurdjieff	Journey to Inaccessible Places	*EG Records (1986)*
R/U	Robert Gass	Pilgrimage	*Spring Hill Music*
R/U	Steven Halpern	Gifts of the Angels	*Inner Peace (1994)*
R/U	Gabrielle Roth	Totem & Refuge	*www.ravenrecording.com*

CHORAL

R/U	**Benedictine Monks**	**Chant**	*Angel*
R/U	**Sound of Light**	**Sound of Light**	*Sound of Light*
U	Voices of Ascension	Beyond Chant	*Delos (1994)*
U	Robert Gass	Songs of Healing	*Spring Hill Music*

WORLD MUSIC

U	**Henri Dikongue**	**C'est la vie (African)**	*www.worldmusic.com/tinder*
U	Boy Ge Mendes	Lagoa (Brazilian)	*www.worldmusic.com/tinder*
S/U	Govi	Andalusian Nights (Flamenco)	*Higher Octave (1999)*
S/U	Buena Vista Social Club	Buena Vista Social Club (Cuban)	*World Circuit*

ELECTRONIC/KEYBOARD/VOCALS

S/U	Robert Miles	Dreamland	*Arista 1996*
R/U	Andreas Vollenveider	Down to the Moon	*Sony*
S/R	Compilation	Euphoria/Chilled	*www.telstar.co.uk*
S/U	Lost at Last	Ocean of Mercy/Lost at Last	*www.lostatlast.com*
S/U	Lisa Gerrard	Duality	*4AD*
S/U	Loreena McKennitt	The Book of Secrets	*Warner Brothers*
S	Soundtrack	Better Living through Circuitry	*www.moonshine.com*
R	Cafe Del Mar	5 & 7	*Mercury Records*
S/R	Compilation	The Chillout Album 1&2	*www.telstar.co.uk*

CLASSICAL

R/U	Compilation	Shadows and Light	*Deutsche Grammophon (1995)*
R/U	Albinoni/Pachelbel	Adagios	*Warner Classics (1996)*
S/U	Dvorak	New World Symphony	*Essential Classics*
R/U	Brahms	Symphony No. 4	*Classical Navigator*
S	J. S. Bach	Brandenburg Concertos	*Pearl*
S	Handel	Water Music Suite, Music for the Royal Fireworks	*Columbia*
S/U	Beethoven	Fourth, Fifth and Ninth Symphonies	*EMI*
S/U	Vivaldi	Four Seasons (Spring and Summer)	*Eloquence*

All these CDs can be ordered on www.naturallyhigh.co.uk, except those which quote website addresses for ordering.

21

SLEEP

A GOOD SNOOZE is the cheapest, safest, most available and most natural high going. According to experts, if you want to be fully alert, cheerful, mentally sharp, creative and energetic all day, you need to spend about 8 hours a night, or one-third of your life, asleep.

'People have no idea how important sleep is to their lives,' says Thomas Roth, Health and Scientific Advisor of the National Sleep Foundation and director of the Sleep Disorders Research Center at Henry Ford Hospital in Detroit. 'Good health demands good sleep. Conversely, lack of sleep and sleep problems have serious, often life-threatening consequences.'[1]

Why do we need so much sleep? Our bodies are governed by dozens of internal clocks that coordinate our inner rhythms in such areas as hormone production, moods, body temperature and energy level. They are regulated by the circadian clock, the cycles of day and night and seasons, governed by the sustainer of life, the Sun. To sustain their dynamic balance, these systems all require that we spend sufficient time sleeping. We are not alone in this. Nearly all animals and even some plants sleep on a regular basis, repairing and rejuvenating themselves during this 'dormant' period.

Just like the over-used stress response, our genetic blueprint for sleep has not evolved quickly enough to keep pace with our emerging 24-hour-a-day lives. Before the electric light bulb extended our days, most people slept an average of 10 hours a night. In the 1950s and 1960s, the average dropped to 8, and it now hovers around 7 and continues to fall. More than 1 in 3 people boast of sleeping 6 hours or less.

Loss of sleep has its price. Even minimal sleep loss makes us less alert and attentive, and more moody and irritable. As our concentration and judgement wane and our ability to perform even simple tasks declines, our true productivity shrinks. At the same time, accident rates increase, as do health problems, in our gastrointestinal, cardiovascular, hormonal and immune systems. Our relationships suffer too. Pointing to our escalating pace of life, work pressures and ageing, many medical specialists now believe sleep disorders to be a major health problem. And disturbed sleep reflects and affects everything else that goes on in our body and mind. The ancient Chinese and other traditional medical systems knew to account for these cycles in both diagnosis and treatment.

REM Sleep: A Chance to Dream

Sleep is a complex and dynamic process with its own rhythms. Sleep labs monitor these patterns through the use of an electroencephalograph or EEG. Electrodes are attached to specific locations on a subject's scalp, and physiological changes are recorded on graph paper in a series of jagged lines. Specialists can tell which stage of sleep someone is in and, by reviewing a full night's recording, whether or not the individual has a normal sleep cycle.

After about half an hour, sleep becomes physically restorative as cells start to repair and rejuvenate. In an hour or so, you shift into the highly active stage called 'REM sleep', characterised by accelerated dreaming and rapid eye movements (REM). Though we may dream in all stages of sleep, dreams occur most frequently in REM sleep and are usually more vivid and emotional than during other stages. For most adults, REM sleep occurs every 90 minutes throughout the night. As the night progresses, REM periods become longer, up to 30 to 45 minutes, and become a dominant part of the sleep cycle. This pattern, with the longer REM period coming at the end of the sleep cycle, offers one of the clearest arguments for getting at least 7 or 8 hours' sleep.

During REM sleep the brain replenishes its supply of neurotransmitters, such as noradrenalin and serotonin, crucial for new learning and retention, as well as mood. The subconscious mind analyses the day's events and processes feelings, an essential activity for mental health. Thus, adequate REM sleep is vital for memory storage, retention, organisation, reorganisation, new learning and emotional balance. In fact, REM sleep is rather like running a clean-up programme on your computer. During the day we generate a lot of open and disconnected circuits, and probably end up with plenty of fragmented and corrupted files. Unless we run our nightly clean-up, the next day our human computer is likely to run slower and less efficiently, to say nothing of the occasional system errors and total crashes we're likely to face.

Recent experiments led by Dr Robert Stickgold at Harvard Medical School demonstrated how we need sleep to retain new learning.[2] The experiments point to a new theory of memory formation involving the interaction between two stages of sleep, one that occurs at the beginning of the night and one that occurs early in the morning. When people learn a new skill, their performance does not improve until after they have had more than 6 and preferably 8 hours of sleep. Without adequate sleep, skills and even new factual information may not get properly encoded into the brain's memory circuits. In fact, a person's intelligence may be less important than a good night's sleep in forming many kinds of memories. Cramming all night before final exams, then, may get you through the next day (on an adrenalin high), but you are likely to forget most of what you learned.

A recent study showed that increased REM sleep time is an excellent mood enhancer. Just think of all the prescriptions written for neurotransmitter-enhancing antidepressants, or sleeping pills, when the underlying problem is actually sleep deprivation. In fact, many of these drugs may actually suppress REM sleep, and reduce available neurotransmitters, thereby aggravating low moods.

You can see now why REM deficiency, sleep deprivation and fatigue often develop into a self-perpetuating cycle:

▶ Decreased sleep reduces REM
▶ Reduced REM prevents rejuvenation
▶ Unrejuvenated, we are more susceptible to stress
▶ Feeling stressed decreases sleep.

Add sleeping pills to the mix, and you accelerate the problem.

Natural Sleep Aids: And So To Bed

Having created a social epidemic of sleep deprivation, we need now to turn away from drugs that basically knock us unconscious, then rob us of our precious restorative REM sleep. Fortunately, we have herbs such as kava, that besides its ability to promote calm and well-being, provides an effective natural treatment for insomnia. Kava seems to work with the body to bring on deep restful sleep without interfering with its natural cycles. Other sleep-promoting herbs include valerian, California poppy, skullcap, hops, and passion flower (see Chapter 4).

Sleep disorders are sometimes linked with lowered brain levels of the neurotransmitter serotonin and its metabolite, melatonin. The herb St John's wort has both serotonin- and melatonin-enhancing effects, making it an excellent sleep regulator. Many of our patients notice that their sleep improves markedly after a few weeks on St John's wort (see Chapter 6). Another choice is 5-hydroxytryptophan, which enhances sleep by increasing serotonin levels (see Chapter 6). Try 50mg 1 hour before bedtime. If that doesn't work, increase to 100mg or a maximum of 200mg.

The hormone melatonin is another important aid to sleep, which is instrumental in establishing our daily rhythms. As we age, our melatonin levels decrease, with the steepest decline occurring after 50. Melatonin supplements may play a role in restoring internal sleeping and waking rhythms, as it works on an underlying physiological cause of sleep disorder. In one study, using melatonin, men and women between the ages of 68 to 80 fell asleep in half their usual time. They also reported their sleep was more refreshing. (Melatonin is available in some countries, but not in the UK.)

If you want to try it, begin with 1mg the first night and, if it works, continue with that dose. If not, increase by 1mg each night, but only up to a 5mg maximum. If you wake up groggy, cut back. Your internal clock should be reset after about 2 weeks, at which point you can discontinue the melatonin. While its popularity has increased due to its possible anti-ageing effects, it is still a hormone, and needs to be appropriately prescribed and monitored.

Taking supplements and sleep aids is only one way of bringing on that moment when, after a long day, with its myriad responsibilities and stresses, you collapse into bed, crawl under the cosy covers, and finally sink into sleep. A good night's sleep is an art that you can learn.

The box below shows you ways of promoting healthy sleeping.

Sleep Exercise

▶ Develop a routine in your sleeping and waking. Irregular bedtimes and waking times is not conducive to a good night's sleep.

▶ Avoid stimulants in the evening and, ideally, throughout the day. They contribute to high cortisol levels in the evening which give your body the wrong message.

▶ Exercise in the evening, which helps 'burn up' the stress hormones of the day, but not within 2 hours of going to bed.

▶ Don't eat late. You need to leave at least 2 hours between dinner and bedtime.

▶ Do something relaxing before bed. This could be listening to music. Some meditative, repetitive music can be used to go to sleep to at a very low volume. If this works for you, the music may soon act as a trigger. Others prefer silence.

▶ Avoid stressful inputs just before bedtime. This includes the news and violent TV programmes.

▶ If you need it, try kava, valerian or 5-HTP. If you wake up in the early hours of the morning and sleep lightly in the morning you may be serotonin-deficient, so 5-HTP can help.

PART FOUR

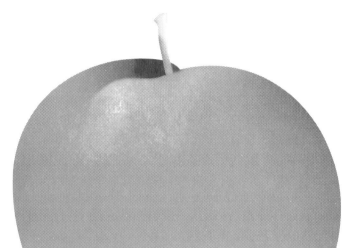

NATURAL HIGHS AT A GLANCE

22

TOP TIPS

I N THE Top Tips that follow, we give you instant programmes to chill out, get an energy boost, improve your mood, sharpen your mind, and/or get connected. As well as following these highly effective action plans, you also need to:

▶ Follow the 'Natural High Basics' diet (page 34) and supplement guidelines.

▶ If applicable, break your dependency to stimulants, cigarettes or tranquillisers (see Appendix, page 275).

▶ Make sure you're not holding on to resolved emotions. If you are even a little bit upset with your mate, for example, a few words of clarification can go a long way towards domestic peace, and even bliss. If you are holding on to work-related upsets, again, clear them either with the person involved, internally, or in a discussion with your partner, a friend, whomever you can get to listen (and preferably, empathise). Holding on to negative emotions is an energy and mood drain, while expressing them helps to dissipate the charge, allowing more energy for positive pursuits, and for feeling high.

Now – on with the Top Tips!

Top Tips for a Natural Chill-out

If you come home from a hard day's work, stressed and in need of chilling out, here's what to do:

▶ Take the following natural relaxants:

Either a 'chill' formula containing kava 60mg (kavalactones), valerian 50mg, hops 100mg, passion flower 100mg, GABA 500mg and taurine 500mg

or kava alone (start with the equivalent of 60 to 75mg of kavalactones).

▶ Do a Vital Energy Exercise (yoga, t'ai chi or *Psychocalisthenics* – see pages 202, 204).

▶ Have a bath with lavender, orange, marjoram and/or chamomile oil in it.

▶ Meditate (see page 207) or listen to biofeedback tapes (see page 212) or do the Breathing Exercise (see page 199).

▶ Put on some relaxing music (see pages 246–7).

▶ Have a massage. Or give yourself a massage (see page 224).

▶ Light your room with candles and/or blue or turquoise light.

▶ Have sex.

▶ Have a nap, if you need it. (Before or after sex – during sex is poor form.)

Top Tips for a Natural Energy Boost

If your 'get up and go' has got up and gone and you need a natural energy boost, here's what to do:

▶ Take the following supplements:

Either an 'energy' formula containing Siberian ginseng 100mg, Asian/American ginseng 100mg, ashwaganda 400mg, reishi mushroom 3000mg, rhodiola 100mg, DLPA 150mg, tyrosine 150mg and pantothenic acid 100mg

or supplement Siberian ginseng (400mg) and some licorice (500mg).

▶ Have a bath or scent your room with lemon, eucalyptus, cinnamon or peppermint (see page 239).

▶ Do some exercise (see page 193).

▶ Do a Vital Energy Exercise such as yoga, t'ai chi or *Psychocalisthenics* (see pages 202, 204).

▶ Put on some stimulating music and boogie to the beat. Close the windows if your neighbours are not heavy metal aficionados (see pages 246–7).

▶ Maximise the light in your room, with natural daylight or full-spectrum lighting.

Top Tips for a Natural Mood Lift

If you're feeling low and need to perk up to get back on track, here's what to do:

▶ Take the following:

   Either a 'mood-boosting' formula containing 5-HTP 50mg, St John's wort 300mg, tyrosine 500mg, DLPA 500mg, SAMe 200mg or TMG 600mg, Niacin (B3) 40mg, pantothenic acid (B5) 100mg, pyridoxine (B6) 20mg, B12 10mcg and folic acid 100mcg

   or try some 5-HTP (starting at 50mg) or some St John's wort (900mg). Remember, though, St John's wort may take a few days or even weeks to kick in; but the wait is worthwhile.

▶ Do some aerobic exercise and/or a Vital Energy Exercise (yoga, t'ai chi or *Psychocalisthenics* – see pages 202, 204).

▶ Do the Light Exercise (see page 232).

▶ Put on some inspiring music, the kind that goes right to your heart and soul (see pages 246–7).

▶ Have a bath or scent your room with bergamot, geranium, petitgrain or neroli oil.

▶ Maximise the light in your room, with natural daylight or full-spectrum lighting.

Top Tips for Natural Mind Enhancement

If your razor-sharp intellect is blunted and your memory is failing you, here's what to do for that extra mental edge:

▶ Take the following:

A 'mind-boosting' formula containing phosphatidyl choline 200mg, DMAE 200mg, pyroglutamate 300mg, phosphatidyl serine 50mg, ginkgo 20mg, vinpocetine 10mg, B complex or B3 50mg, B5 (pantothenic acid) 50mg, B6 50mg, B12 50mcg, folic acid 400mcg topped up by what's in your multivitamin.

plus a fish oil supplement giving 500mg of DHA/EPA – or eat fish three times a week.

▶ Do some aerobic exercise. It will oxygenate your brain, raise endorphins and, as an added bonus, burn some fat.

▶ Have a bath or scent your room with lemon, eucalyptus, cinnamon or peppermint (see page 239).

▶ Put on some stimulating music (see pages 246–7).

▶ Maximise the light in your room, with natural daylight or full-spectrum lighting.

Top Tips for Getting Connected Naturally

If you're feeling dis-connected and you've lost your sparkle, here's how to get reconnected and back in the flow:

▶ Take the following:

Either a 'connector nutrient' formula providing 5-HTP 50mg, SAMe 200mg or TMG 600mg, kava 100mg, sceletium 100mg, B complex (B3 50mg, B5 or pantothenic acid 50mg, B6 50mg, B12 50mcg, folic acid 400mcg) topped up by what's in your multivitamin

or try some SAMe (start with 200mg), 5-HTP (start with 50mg) or kava (start with 60 to 75 mg of a standardised extract).

▶ Put on some inspiring music (see pages 246–7).

▶ Do a Vital Energy Exercise (yoga, t'ai chi or *Psychocalisthenics* – see pages 202, 204).

▶ Meditate (see page 207) or listen to the biofeedback tapes (see page 212).

▶ Have, or give, a massage (see page 224).

▶ Have great sex.

▶ Have a bath with or scent your room with lavender.

▶ Light your room with candles or violet, magenta or blue light.

23

A–Z OF NATURAL HIGHS

Acetyl-L-carnitine

▶ mind and memory booster

How it works: Fuel for the brain, helps make acetylcholine and acts as an antioxidant.

Positive effects: Improves mood and mental performance.

Cautions: Not recommended for those with diabetes or liver or kidney disease.

How much?: 250–1500mg, away from food.

Ashwaganda (*Withania somnifera*)

▶ stimulant

How it works: Acts as an adaptogen, stabilising cortisol levels.

Positive effects: Energising, calming, reduces high cortisol levels, enhances libido, memory and cognition.

Cautions: None.

How much?: 300mg two to three times daily.

B vitamins

▶ **stimulant**

▶ **mood enhancer**

▶ **mind and memory booster**

▶ **connector**

How they work: Turn glucose into energy in neurons, co-factors for making neurotransmitters, help transport oxygen, protect the brain from toxins and oxidants, vital for enzymes that control the chemistry of connection, act as methyl group donors and acceptors.

Positive effects: Raise IQ, improve energy, memory, mood, concentration. B vitamins also help prevent unpleasant hallucinations experienced in some types of schizophrenia.

Cautions: None in sensible doses. Excess B3 and B6 (above 1000mg a day) can have adverse effects. B3 as niacin acts as a vasodilator, improving circulation and causing blushing at doses above 50mg.

How much?: For B1, B2, B3, B6: 50–100mg. B5: 50–500mg. B12:10–1000mcg. Folic acid: 400–1000mcg.

Choline

▶ **mind and memory booster**

How it works: Precursor for the neurotransmitter acetylcholine and part of structure of neuronal membranes.

Positive effects: More alert, clear-headed, better memory and concentration, improved brain development during pregnancy in rats.

Cautions None.

How much?: Lecithin 5–10g (tablespoon) or hi-phosphatidyl choline lecithin 2.5–5g (heaped teaspoon) or phosphatidyl choline 1–2g or choline 300–600mg.

DHA

▶ mood enhancer

▶ mind and memory booster

How it works: Building material for neuronal membranes and neurotransmitter receptor sites, and increases acetylcholine and serotonin levels.

Positive effects: Improves learning, memory and mood in both depression, manic depression, dyslexia and dyspraxia.

Cautions: None. DHA does help reduce blood clotting. High doses should not be taken if you are on blood-thinning medication.

How much?: 250-500mg a day as a fish oil supplement or eat oily fish three times a week.

(See also Omega-3 fats.)

DMAE

▶ mind and memory booster

How it works: Precursor for choline which crosses readily into the brain, hence helping to make acetylcholine.

Positive effects: More alert, improves concentration and reduces anxiety, improves learning and attention span, normalises brain-wave patterns.

Cautions: Too much can overstimulate and is therefore not recommended for those diagnosed with schizophrenia, mania or epilepsy. Lower the dose if you find you experience insomnia.

How much?: 100–300mg, taken in the morning or midday, not in the evening.

EPA

▶ mood enhancer

▶ mind and memory booster

How it works: Precursor for prostaglandins, which influence mood and behaviour and probably neurotransmitter balance.

Positive effects: Helps restore normal behaviour in mental illness. May affect mood and memory.

Cautions: None. EPA does help reduce blood clotting. High doses should not be taken if you are on blood-thinning medication.

How much?: 250–500mg a day as a fish oil supplement or eat oily fish three times a week.

(See also Omega-3 fats.)

GABA

▶ relaxant

How it works: Calming neurotransmitter, enhances natural GABA activity which counteracts stress hormones.

Positive effect: Reduces anxiety, insomnia and tension.

Cautions: Nausea and vomiting at high doses.

How much?: 500–1000mg twice daily after meals.

Ginkgo biloba

▶ mind and memory booster

How it works: Improves circulation, acts as an antioxidant.

Positive effects: Improves mood, memory, concentration and energy.

Cautions: Blood thinner: use with caution if already taking blood-thinning medication. Rare side effects of headaches, nausea or nosebleeds have been reported at high doses.

How much?: 60–240mg a day of a standardised extract providing 24 per cent flavonoids, taken in two or three divided doses.

Ginseng – Siberian and Asian

▶ stimulant

How it works: Acts as adaptogen, supporting the adrenal glands.

Positive effects: Enhances the body's response to stress, decreasing feelings of anxiety and stress and increasing immediate energy (stimulant). Restores vitality, energy and endurance over time (tonic). Increases mental and physical performance.

Cautions: None for Siberian ginseng. For Asian ginseng, possible menstrual abnormalities and breast tenderness. Over-use can cause over-stimulation, including insomnia in sensitive individuals. Take a 1-month break after taking ginseng for 3 months.

How much?: For Siberian ginseng 200–400mg daily; for Asian ginseng 100–200mg daily of a standardised extract containing 4 to 7 per cent ginsenosides.

5-HTP

▶ mood enhancer

▶ connector

How it works: Precursor for the neurotransmitter serotonin and some tryptamines.

Positive effects: Improves mood, induces relaxation, healthy appetite control, healthy sleep-wake patterns, emotional stability, dreaming and visioning. An effective antidepressant.

Cautions: Nausea and GI problems in high doses. It is inadvisable to take both 5-HTP and SSRI antidepressants except under medical guidance.

How much?: 100–300mg for the treatment of depression or insomnia, 100mg as natural connector or mood enhancer, best taken as 50mg twice daily. If used for insomnia take an hour before bedtime.

Kava

▶ relaxant

▶ connector

How it works: Calms the limbic system, the emotional centre of the brain and relaxes muscles, likely through an indirect action on GABA receptors. Kava has chemical similarities to MDMA.

Positive effects: It is able to relax both muscles and emotions, reducing excessive mental 'chatter', increasing mental focus, and expanding overall awareness, connection and empathy. Also promotes good sleep. An effective anti-anxiety agent and muscle relaxant. The muscle-relaxing effects make it particularly useful in treating headaches, backaches and other tension-related pain.

Cautions: Do not drive or operate heavy machinery after use; do not mix with alcohol, as the two substances seem to potentiate each other; do not take while using benzodiazepine tranquillisers.

How much?: As a relaxant, the normal dosage is approximately 60–75mg of kavalactones; as a bedtime sedative, 120–200mg; as a connector, 150–500mg.

Licorice (*Glycyrrhiza glabra*)

▶ stimulant

How it works: Prevents the breakdown of cortisol, thereby raising cortisol levels.

Positive effects: Improves adrenal function if exhausted, and raises low blood pressure if adrenally exhausted.

Cautions: Can raise blood pressure in susceptible individuals. Not recommended for those with raised cortisol levels.

How much?: 500mg twice a day, morning and midday, not in the evening.

Omega-3 fats – EPA and DHA

▶ mood enhancer

▶ mind and memory booster

How they work: Building material for neuronal membranes and neurotransmitter receptor sites, enhancing neural transmission and increasing serotonin levels.

Positive effects: Improve learning, memory and mood in both depression, manic depression, dyslexia and dyspraxia.

Cautions: None.

How much?: 500–1000mg a day as a fish oil supplement or eat oily fish three times a week.

DL-phenylalanine (DLPA)

▶ **stimulant**

▶ **mood enhancer**

How it works: Precursor for tyrosine which converts to dopamine, adrenalin and noradrenalin.

Positive effects: Enhances mood, promotes energy, relieves pain and controls appetite.

Cautions: Can be too stimulating, generating anxiety, high blood pressure or insomnia; should not be taken by phenylketonurics. Not recommended for those with a history of mania or mental illness.

How much?: 500–1000mg of DLPA on an empty stomach first thing in the morning.

Phosphatidyl serine

▶ **mind and memory booster**

How it works: Building material for neuronal membranes and neurotransmitter receptor sites.

Positive effects: Improves mood, memory, stress resistance, learning and concentration.

Cautions: None.

How much?: 100–300mg a day.

Pyroglutamate

▶ mind and memory booster

How it works: Increases acetylcholine production and improves reception.

Positive effects: Improves memory, cognitive function and concentration, coordination and reaction time, and improves communication between right and left hemispheres of the brain.

Cautions: None.

How much?: 400–1000mg.

Reishi mushroom (*Ganodermum lucidum*)

▶ stimulant

How it works: Acts as an adaptogen, stabilising adrenal hormones.

Positive effects: Both calming and energising.

Cautions: None.

How much: In tincture form (20 per cent), 10ml three times day; as tablets 1000mg, one to three tablets three times a day.

Rhodiola (*Rhodiola rosea*)

▶ stimulant

How it works: Acts as an adaptogen, stabilising adrenal hormones and promoting serotonin production.

Positive effects: Improves concentration, stress resistance, physical performance and mood. Boosts immunity.

Cautions: None.

How much?: 200–300mg daily of a standardised extract, with meals.

SAMe (s-adenosyl-methionine)

▶ mood enhancer

▶ connector

How it works: Naturally occurring molecule, donates methyl group in manufacture of neurotransmitters, as well as DNA. It therefore acts as a catalyst for producing a wide range of key brain chemicals, including DMT, serotonin, dopamine and noradrenalin. SAMe is produced from the amino acid methionine. Also important in liver detoxification.

Positive effects: Enhances neurotransmitter activity, acts as a natural antidepressant, stimulant and mood enhancer. Generally improves energy, mental clarity, emotional balance and mood, promoting natural connection.

Cautions: In some people higher doses of SAMe have been known to induce nausea. Taking SAMe with food reduces this possibility, but is less effective from the point of view of absorption. Very high doses may lead to irritability, anxiety and insomnia. SAMe's antidepressant activity may lead to the manic phase in individuals with bipolar disorder (manic depression), so such individuals should be monitored carefully.

How much?: 200mg twice daily, on an empty stomach, increasing gradually to a maximum of 1600mg a day if needed.

Sceletium

▶ mood enhancer

▶ connector

How it works: Appears to enhance serotonin activity, the mood-enhancing neurotransmitter, and balance dopamine, adrenalin and noradrenalin; there is still much that is unknown about its effects on the brain.

Positive effects: Lessens depression, tension and anxiety, promotes a sense of connection. Associated with insights, heightened sensory perception and improving meditation. Also reduces addictive cravings.

Cautions: In very large doses can have euphoric effects, followed by sedation. No reported toxicity.

How much?: As a mood enhancer, the normal dosage is 50–100mg; as a connector, 100–200mg.

St John's wort

▶ mood enhancer

How it works: It probably inhibits re-uptake of neurotransmitters serotonin, noradrenalin and dopamine, and enhances GABA activity as well.

Positive effects: Mood-enhancing; both antidepressant, anti-anxiety and sleep-enhancing.

Cautions: May cause allergic reactions, rashes, gastrointestinal problems, sun sensitivity in susceptible individuals. Can cause anxiety, or insomnia in certain individuals if taken too close to bedtime. It can reduce the potency of protease inhibitors (for AIDS) or cyclosporin (an organ transplant immune suppressant), digoxin (heart medication) or even, possibly, birth-control pills. There is no proof as yet for this last one – it is theoretical only. It has not been researched sufficiently to recommend its use in pregnancy and breast-feeding.

How much?: 300mg of an extract of 0.3 per cent hypericin, starting with one or two capsules/tablets in the morning with breakfast. If there is no change after a week, add a third dose at lunch. You can also take it as two doses of 450mg each, or take your entire daily dose in the morning, since the effect lasts for a long time.

Taurine

▶ relaxant

How it works: Enhances GABA activity, the calming neurotransmitter.

Positive effect: Reduces anxiety, irritability, insomnia, migraine, alcoholism, obsessions and depression.

Cautions: Drug interactions.

How much?: 500–1000mg twice daily.

L-tryptophan

▶ mood enhancer

▶ connector

How it works: Precursor for the neurotransmitter serotonin, DMT and all tryptamines. Can be converted into niacin (vitamin B3).

Positive effects: Promotes relaxation, elevated mood, deep sleep, healthy sleep-wake patterns, emotional stability, dreaming and visioning. L-tryptophan is an effective antidepressant.

Cautions: Nausea and gastrointestinal upset problems in high doses. There is a theoretical risk of 'serotonin syndrome' if taking both tryptophan and SSRI antidepressants, so it is inadvisable to take both except under medical guidance.

How much?: 1000–3000mg for the treatment of depression or insomnia, 1000mg as a mood enhancer or natural connector. Best absorbed away from food or with a carbohydrate snack, such as a piece of fruit. If used for insomnia take an hour before bedtime. Best taken with B vitamins.

Tyrosine

▶ stimulant

How it works: Precursor to stimulating neurotransmitters dopamine, adrenalin, noradrenalin and thyroid hormone, thyroxine.

Positive effects: Enhances mood, promotes energy and motivation, supports healthy thyroid function.

Cautions: Hypertension in those susceptible. Should not be taken by phenylketonurics. Not recommended for those with a history of mania or mental illness.

How much?: 500–1000mg on an empty stomach first thing in the morning.

Valerian

▶ relaxant

How it works: Enhances GABA activity.

Positive effects: Reduces anxiety, insomnia and tension.

Cautions: Potentiates sedative drugs, including muscle relaxants and antihistamines, so it is not recommended to take both.

How much?: For relaxation, 50–100mg two to three times daily; for sleep, 150–300mg about 45 minutes before bedtime.

Vinpocetine

▶ **mind and memory booster**

How it works: Improves blood flow and circulation to the brain.

Positive effects: Improves cognitive performance. Potentially helpful in epilepsy.

Cautions: None reported.

How much?: 10–40mg a day.

APPENDIX
Breaking the Cycle
of Addiction

How to Quit Smoking

The first thing we want to say is: you can quit. This statement might seem counterintuitive if you've tried and failed, or can't imagine ever stopping. And there's no doubt that nicotine is addictive stuff.

In fact, it's more addictive than heroin, and this is what makes cigarettes hard to quit. Those little tubes contain not only nicotine but 16 other cancer-producing chemicals, as well. Nicotine also produces a substantial effect even in small doses, and in large amounts acts as a sedative. This is its attraction: on the one hand, it can give you a lift; on the other, it can calm you down. Before a meal it can stop you feeling hungry; after a meal it can stop you from feeling drowsy.

All of these effects are down to nicotine's action on adrenal hormones, blood sugar and brain chemicals. By strictly following the advice given in Chapter 3, 'Natural High Basics', the craving for cigarettes will diminish. And that's because you'll stabilise your blood sugar and hormone levels.

So, before you even begin to try to quit cigarettes, we recommend following these diet and supplement guidelines strictly for 2 months, preferably with the guidance and support of a clinical nutritionist, until you no longer consume any other stimulants (such as tea, coffee and chocolate or sugar). Instead you'll be eating small, frequent meals, with an emphasis on foods containing slow-releasing carbohydrates combined with foods rich in proteins.

Breaking all the habits

The average smoker is addicted not only to nicotine, but also to smoking when tired, hungry or upset, on waking, after a meal with a drink and so on. Before you actually give up smoking altogether, it's best to break these mental associations.

At first don't attempt to change your smoking habits. Just keep a diary for a week, writing down every situation in which you smoke, how you feel before and how you feel after smoking. You can copy the style below to record your 1-week smoking diary.

SMOKING DIARY		
Day _ _ _ _ _ _		
Time Situation	**Feeling Before**	**Feeling After**
9am With coffee	*Tired*	*Awake*

When the week is up, add up how many cigarettes you smoke in each situation. Your list might look something like this:

▶ With a hot drink – 16

▶ After a meal – 6

▶ With alcohol – 4

▶ Difficult situation – 4

▶ After sex – 3

Now set yourself fortnightly targets. For the first 2 weeks, smoke as much as you like whenever you like but not when you drink a hot drink. For the next 2 weeks, smoke as much as you like whenever you like but not when you drink a hot drink, or within 30 minutes of finishing a meal. Continue like this until, when you smoke, all you do is smoke, without the associated habits.

This will be tremendously helpful for you when you quit. Most people start again because the phone rings with a problem, someone brings in a coffee, offers you a cigarette … and before you know it you're smoking.

Reduce your nicotine load

Now it's time to reduce your nicotine load gradually. Week by week, switch to a brand that contains less nicotine, until what you smoke contains no more than 2mg per cigarette. In addition to the supplements recommended in Chapter 3, 'Natural High Basics', supplementing 1000mg of vitamin C, 100mcg of chromium and 50mg of niacin with each meal should help reduce your cravings. You may experience a blushing sensation when first taking niacin. This is harmless and usually occurs 15 to 30 minutes after taking it, and lasts for about 15 minutes. The blushing is less likely to occur if you take niacin with a meal, and will diminish and, in most cases, stop completely if you take 50mg three times a day.

Increasing the alkaline balance of your body helps reduce cravings: a way to achieve this is by eating a diet that is high in fruit, vegetables and seeds. In addition, consider supplementing calcium (600mg) and magnesium (400mg) daily, as these are alkaline minerals and help to neutralise excess acidity.

Whenever you feel the need for nicotine, first eat an apple or a pear. This will raise a low blood sugar level, which is often the factor that triggers such a craving.

Regular exercise also helps, so this is a great time to sign up at your local gym, start jogging or learn psychocalisthenics (see Chapter 12).

Now reduce the number of cigarettes you are smoking until you smoke no more than five cigarettes a day, each with a nicotine content of 2mg or less. If you wish, stop smoking and replace with nicotine gum as an intermediate step. (Nicotine gum comes in two strengths – 4mg and 2mg.)

You want to be down to a maximum of 10mg of nicotine a day before quitting – that is, five pieces of 2mg nicotine gum, or five 2mg nicotine cigarettes.

Time to quit

It's now time to quit. Give yourself all the support you can get. Make sure your friends and work colleagues know so they can help by not trying to stress you out or overreacting if you are not at your best. It's great to have a buddy you can talk to whenever you crave nicotine. They can help you strengthen your resolve.

The sensations you have when withdrawing from nicotine are a direct effect of its action on your blood sugar, adrenal hormone levels and key chemicals in the brain. It is incredibly helpful to follow a really good nutritional programme during the first month after quitting. Make sure you always have a good breakfast, lunch and dinner and have low-GI snacks (see Chapter 3, 'Natural High Basics' page 26) available during the day when your blood sugar levels dip. You may also find it helpful to take a 5-hydroxytryptophan (5-HTP) supplement. This is an amino acid that the body converts into serotonin, an important brain chemical that controls mood. Nicotine withdrawal tends to lower serotonin levels, which leaves you depressed and irritable. You can prevent this from happening by supplementing 200mg of 5-HTP, which is available in health-food stores. 5-HTP is best absorbed if you take it away from protein foods and with carbohydrate foods, so either take it on a empty stomach, or with a piece of fruit. And because serotonin levels rise at night promoting a good night's sleep, the best time to take your 5-HTP is an hour before bed.

Another useful aid during the first month is licorice, which promotes the action of adrenal hormones. Since nicotine acts as an adrenal stimulant, additional adrenal support can be helpful during the withdrawal phase. Licorice is either available as a supplement or as a bar. The bar we'd recommend is Panda licorice, which is sweetened with molasses rather than sugar. As far as supplements are concerned, the amount to take is 1 to 2g powdered root, or 2 to 4ml fluid extract three times a day. Check the manufacturer's instructions, as potencies can vary. Licorice should be avoided or used with caution by people with high blood pressure – visit a herbalist to be sure.

Detox your body

One factor that helps to reduce cravings is boosting the body's ability to detoxify and eliminate chemicals, including nicotine. There are five things you can do to speed up this process: exercise, sweating, drinking plenty of water and supplementing vitamin C and niacin. Put these all together, and you've got a winning formula for rapid detoxification.

If you have access to a sauna or steam room, here's what to do. (Most gyms have one or the other. This is a great opportunity to enrol in a regular exercise programme.)

▶ Take 1g of vitamin C and 100mg of niacin.

▶ Go for a run or undertake any cardiovascular exercise that raises your pulse rate and stimulates circulation.

▶ Once you start blushing as a consequence of the niacin, enter the sauna or steam room.

▶ The sauna should never be at a temperature above 27°C (80°F).

▶ Take in a litre of water and keep drinking it at regular intervals.

Do this for half an hour every day. This routine is *not* recommended for those with a history of cardiovascular disease, however, except with medical supervision. While no danger is anticipated or reported, the combination of exercise, niacin and saunas is a substantial stimulation to circulation, and hence cellular detoxification, which is the purpose of this routine.

Are You a Stimulant Addict?

Do you ever buy sweets and hide the wrappers so other people won't know? Do you swoon at the dessert menu in restaurants and always take a mint or two on the way out? How much do you think about and look forward to that cup of coffee in the morning or in the break? How important to you is that drink after work? How secret are you about the amount you smoke? Have you become a coffee connoisseur, side-stepping the issue of addiction by focusing on your hobby of sampling yet another caffeinated offering? This kind of relationship to stimulants, often cloaked in the attitude that these are just the normal pleasures of life, is indicative of an underlying chemical imbalance that depletes your energy and peace of mind.

Even if this sounds like you, you'll still need to assess, for yourself, your current relationship to stimulants. All you need to do is keep a daily diary, just for 3 days. Mark down how much and when you consume coffee, tea, chocolate, sugar or something sweet, cigarettes or alcohol. And note how intensely you crave them.

Hint for handling cravings: take a 500mg capsule of L-glutamine, open it, and pour the powdered contents under your tongue. It is absorbed quickly, and gives a pick-up similar to that of your longed-for stimulant. You can also take a 500mg capsule several times a day, between meals, to prevent cravings. Adding DL-phenylalanine, 500mg, two to three times daily will give you an energy boost as well.

You don't need them

Stimulants are energy's greatest enemy. Even though stimulants can create energy in the short term, the long-term effect is always bad. The same is true for stress. So the first step to beating stress and fatigue is to cut out, or cut down on, stimulants. That means, as we've noted, coffee, tea, chocolate, sugar and refined foods, cigarettes, cola drinks and alcohol.

Go cold turkey, and quit consuming these stimulants for 1 month. Notice what happens on withdrawal. The more damage stimulants are doing to you, the greater the withdrawal effect. (Fortunately, by eating slow-releasing carbohydrates and taking energy nutrients as supplements, you can minimise withdrawal symptoms which usually last no more that 4 days.) Then start again, and notice what happens with your first tea, coffee, hit. of sugar and chocolate. You'll experience what Hans Selye (who described the general adaptation syndrome, see the figure on page 43) called the 'initial response' – in other words, a true response to these powerful chemicals: pounding head, hyperactive mind, fast heart-beat and insomnia, followed by extreme drowsiness. Keep on the stimulants and you will adapt – that's phase 2. Keep doing this long enough and eventually you hit exhaustion – phase 3. This happens for everybody. The only variance is how long it will take you to get to the 'exhaustion' phase.

Recovery is not only possible, it's usually rapid. Most people feel substantially more energy and ability to cope with stress within 30 days of quitting stimulants with nutritional support. Remember that decaffeinated coffee still contains stimulants.

The painless way to cut out stimulants

You may have scoffed at the idea of cutting out all stimulants for a month. This would be at least stressful for many people, and just about impossible for some. If this sounds like you, your first step is to find out which stimulants are most important to you. Look at your habits. Which substance, if any, do you have in one form or other several times a day? Which do you use as a pick-me-up, perhaps to get you out of bed in the morning or when your energy is flagging during the day? Which would you find the hardest to stop completely for a month?

Although you may intend to stop them for ever, in reality it is a lot easier to take it one step at a time. So start by picking one stimulant (other than cigarettes) you use frequently. Could you realistically cut it out for a month only? If not, what could you reduce your intake to? Write this down and stick to it. Set yourself similar targets for no more than three stimulants. Sometimes they overlap. For example, if you use coffee, sugar and chocolate, but can't stand coffee without sugar, then cutting out sugar automatically means no chocolate and no coffee.

Here are some tips to help you get started.

Sugar

Sugar is an acquired taste. Although we are born with a liking for sweet things, research has shown that only those who are fed sweets and sweet foods as children like high levels of sweetness. So as you gradually cut down the level of sweetness in *all* the food you eat, you will soon get accustomed to the taste. You'll need to reduce the amount of sugar you have in hot drinks and food, eat less dried fruit, and dilute the fruit juice you drink. When you want something sweet, have a piece of fruit. Sweeten cereals and desserts with fruit, and if you're really desperate have a sugar-free fruit and nut bar from your local health-food store. Don't use sugar substitutes. These may not raise your blood sugar levels, but neither do they allow you to change your habits.

It takes about a month for a preference for less sweet foods to kick in. Let your taste buds be the judge of how sweet a food is – but do check the labels for all those disguised forms of sugar.

Coffee

Coffee is strongly addictive. It takes, on average, 4 days to break the habit. During these days you may experience headaches and grogginess. These are a strong reminder of how bad coffee really is for you. Decaffeinated coffee is only mildly better. The most popular coffee alternatives are Caro, Bamboo, Yannoh, Barleycup and Symington's Dandelion Coffee. When you have been off coffee for a month you may decide the occasional cup would be nice. Have this as a treat, perhaps when you eat out, not as a pick-me-up.

Tea

Tea is not as bad for you as coffee, unless you like your tea well stewed. Start by decreasing the strength of your tea, perhaps using a smaller cup or teapot. Tea has such a strong flavour that you can literally dip a tea bag in for a few seconds and still have a strong-tasting drink. Use Luaka tea, a good-quality Ceylon tea that is naturally low in tannin and caffeine. The most popular caffeine-free alternatives are herb teas such as Celestial Seasonings or Yogi Teas. Red Bush (or Rooibosch) tea is good with milk and has a taste closer to 'normal' tea. Green tea isn't caffeine-free but it has much less than regular tea and has other health benefits.

Chocolate

Chocolate contains both sugar and chocolate. Start by switching to chocolate- and sugar-free snacks from your local health-food store or Panda licorice bars. Then, cut these out too, keeping them strictly for emergencies. Eat fresh fruit instead if you feel you need something sweet.

Alcohol

It is all to easy to over-indulge in alcohol because of its role in social interaction. Start by limiting the times you have alcohol. For example, don't drink at lunchtime. You'll certainly work better in the afternoon. Limit what you drink. For example, stick to wine, avoiding beer or spirits. Limit how much you drink by setting yourself a weekly target – for example, seven glasses of wine a week. This allows you to have quite a few at that party on Saturday night and compensate by having little throughout the proceeding week. Ideally, cut it out completely for at least the first 2 weeks. If you find this hard to do, take a close look at your drinking habits and, if necessary, seek professional help.

To sum up – here are some practical steps for breaking addictions to stress and stimulants:

▶ Identify which stimulants that you are addicted to.

▶ Find which substitutes you like the most, and avoid or considerably reduce your intake of stimulants until they are no longer a daily requirement.

▶ Notice your patterns of stressful behaviour and replace these with a more positive way of responding.

Coming Off Tranquillisers

If you take anti-anxiety drugs, you have a lot of company. In Britain, more than 5 million prescriptions for benzodiazepines such as Valium are written out every year, while almost 4 million Americans take them every day, often for years. Two-thirds of benzodiazepine prescriptions are written by family practitioners, and the remainder by psychiatrists. Research in the late 1970s and early 1980s showed that when taken at the usually prescribed doses, dependence on them can occur after only 1 to 2 weeks.[1] With the increasing recognition of widespread abuse and dependency problems, the number of prescriptions for benzodiazepines in the US gradually dropped from a high of 87 million in 1973 to 55 million in 1981.

This dip, however, was temporary, as a phenomenally aggressive marketing campaign for the introduction of Xanax in the late 1980s reversed the slide in popularity. With this new drug leading the way, prescriptions of all psychoactive medications, including benzodiazepines, again began to climb. Were people actually becoming more depressed and anxious, or were the drugs companies simply doing a better job of selling? While the former could be true, what's now certain is that the companies were, in fact, becoming more aggressive and persuasive in marketing these drugs. (For an excellent examination of these issues, read Edward Drummond's *Overcoming Anxiety Without Tranquillisers*.[2])

As addictive as heroin

Although benzodiazepines suppress the symptoms of anxiety for a few hours, they do not treat underlying causes, and the anxiety returns as soon as the drug wears off. Moreover, there is a 'rebound effect' where the individual experiences even worse symptoms than they started with as a result of chemical dependency. Often, the person develops tolerance, meaning that even higher doses are needed for the same anti-anxiety effect. These factors – withdrawal and tolerance – describe an addiction that can be as difficult as heroin to break. A combination of physical and emotional dependency develops, and protection is not afforded by limiting to 'occasional' use. Ignoring the warning that they are meant to be taken for only weeks at a time, overburdened doctors may continue to renew a prescription for many months or even years.

Consider Jan's story:

A 32-year-old secretary for an insurance company, Jan had been in a car accident two years before I (Hyla) saw her. Another car had hit her from behind with some force. She sustained a variety of injuries, including a shattered kneecap and whiplash, which left her with headaches and neck pain. The accident jarred her emotionally as well. During her week-long hospital stay, she was given Valium as a muscle relaxant and anti-anxiety agent, and Restoril for sleep. The Restoril was understandable, as sleeping in a hospital can be difficult. In time, her injuries healed, but she was left with intermittent neck pain, relieved to some degree by Valium.

Jan was unable to end her dependence on Valium and Restoril. Her attempts to discontinue the medications were met with unbearable insomnia, followed by fatigue and an inability to function. She was hooked, and her doctor continued to renew her prescriptions. She noticed herself becoming absent-minded, not remembering where she had put things in the house, forgetting appointments, and becoming increasingly tired and depressed. She had long since quit her job, unable to cope with any additional responsibilities. Life was bleak, and since the accident, she had a lingering fear of driving. She spent more and more time at home, doing less and less. Her concerned husband brought her to see a psychiatrist, who prescribed an antidepressant. But this had little effect.

Jan was experiencing just about every side effect of the benzodiazepines: poor memory, confusion, depression, lack of coordination and drowsiness. This daytime sedation and mental confusion can, like alcohol ingestion, lead to traffic accidents.[3] Another problem is 'ataxia', a loss of balance – especially problematic when it occurs in the elderly –which can lead to falls and hip fractures.[4]

As Jan discovered, the chronic use of benzodiazepine can actually increase anxiety and depression. This can lead to a narrowing of focus and even total withdrawal and isolation. This may be a slow, insidious process, and, like Jane, you may not think to attribute it to the use of the drug. The resulting depression is often treated with more antidepressants, rather than eliminating the source of the problem by stopping the benzodiazepine itself. This locks you into a vicious cycle, from which you may feel there's no escape.

Minimising withdrawal symptoms with natural remedies

Coming off benzodiazepines has its own hazards. There are several withdrawal effects including insomnia, anxiety, irritability, sweating, blurred vision, diarrhoea, tremors, mental impairment and headaches. Abrupt withdrawal from high doses can lead to seizures or even death.[5] Fortunately, a gradual programme of withdrawal coupled with natural remedies such as kava and valerian can ease and shorten the transition phase.

This is just what I (Hyla) prescribed for Jan. Besides much-needed psychotherapy, I recommended kava and valerian. This not only helped her with anxiety and insomnia, but relieved her lingering neck pain as well. A few visits to a chiropractor completed her recovery. Before long, Jan was able to return to work, at a better job, and her husband thanked me for 'giving me my wife back!'.

Never go it alone

Your ideal withdrawal programme has to be tailored to your circumstances – the amount of the drug taken, length of use and your unique physiology. It takes months to get off these drugs completely, and professional support and guidance are essential.

As we've said, valerian (see page 62) is a great help in the process of withdrawal. A GABA enhancer, it will have similar actions to the drug, but is much gentler and doesn't have the same addictive potential. The same is true for kava (see page 57). You gradually reduce the tranquilliser dose while increasing that of either (or both) valerian and kava. They each have their own actions and 'feel', so the choice depends on how well they're doing the job.

A word of caution. Since benzodiazepines, kava and valerian all enhance GABA, the combination of the herbs with tranquilliser drugs can make the drugs' effects more potent. This point of caution is made by the German government's Commission E Report, a common reference manual on the use of herbal medicines. It recommends care when combining kava with any psychoactive substance, which would include benzodiazepines. For this reason, valerian and kava should be viewed in the same way as any medicine, and taken in carefully scheduled doses as part of the medically supervised withdrawal programme. In other words, you should not just add them in yourself. It is also helpful to add supplements that support the liver's ability to detoxify these drugs, such as milk thistle (*Silymarin silibum*), a liver-enhancing herb that helps to speed up the metabolism of tranquillisers.

Generally, as we decrease the tranquilliser dose, we gradually increase the amount of kava and valerian, replacing the drug with the herbs. Since the herbs are not addictive and do not build tolerance, the person doesn't have to be weaned off them later.

The dose range for valerian is 50 to 100mg two to three times daily. For kava we recommend 60 to 120mg of kavalactones two to three times daily, modified according to where you are in the detox process. If combining the two, take into consideration the addictive effect of the two herbs and adjust these doses accordingly. You also need 60mg of milk thistle twice a day to help along the detoxification process.

To Break An Addiction

To sum up, here are some practical steps to take to break addiction to tranquillisers and minimise symptoms of withdrawal:

▶ Get professional support and guidance.

▶ Deal with psychological issues with the guidance of a psychotherapist.

▶ Start with milk thistle to support the liver, then gradually reduce the tranquilliser dose, under professional guidance, and replace with valerian and kava.

▶ When withdrawal symptoms are gone, reduce the dose of valerian and/or kava.

▶ Follow the dietary guidelines in Chapter 3, 'Natural High Basics', throughout the process.

GLOSSARY

Acetylcholine A stimulating neurotransmitter, associated with memory, mental alertness, learning ability and concentration. Acetylcholine deficiency can lead to memory loss, depression, mood disorders, and possibly even Alzheimer's disease. It is also the neurotransmitter at all nerve-muscle cell junctions that allows skeletal muscles to contract, controlling movement, coordination and muscle tone.

Addiction A pattern of compulsive consumption of a substance, with the need for increased doses over time to maintain the same effect (tolerance), and the appearance of unpleasant symptoms, which disappear when it is reinstated (withdrawal).

Adrenalin (epinephrine in the US) A stimulating neurotransmitter associated with motivation, drive, energy, stimulation and the stress response. Produced by the adrenal glands, it is also classified as a hormone, which is a chemical messenger produced by the glands of the endocrine system.

Amino acid The building blocks of protein. Plants and animals assemble amino acids to make proteins that form different substances such as hormones, neurotransmitters and building materials for the body, such as muscle or skin.

Dendrite Nerve cells (neurons) connect to each other with branches known as dendrites. A neuron can have up to 20,000 dendrites networking with other neurons.

Dopamine A stimulating neurotransmitter associated with pleasure, alertness, concentration and euphoria. Adrenalin and noradrenalin are both made from dopamine.

Downregulation The shutting down of neurotransmitter receptor sites as a consequence of over-stimulation, resulting in the need for increased doses of a substance over time to maintain the same effect (tolerance).

Endorphins A popular term for substances known as 'opiate peptides', which includes enkephalins and dynorphins. These are associated with pleasure, orgasm, euphoria and pain relief. Endorphins are the brain's own natural opiates: they bind to a specific opiate receptor, reducing pain and promoting mild euphoria, such as 'runner's high'.

GABA (gamma-amino-butyric acid) An inhibitory neurotransmitter, associated with relaxation. It has a quieting or dampening effect on the central nervous system, and controls the release of dopamine in the reward centre of the brain.

Monoamine oxidase inhibitor (MAOI) A type of antidepressant drug that inhibits the enzyme, monoamine oxidase, that breaks down neurotransmitters, thereby having the effect of keeping more neurotransmitters in action.

Myelin sheath The insulating layer or membrane around a nerve cell (neuron), made largely out of phospholipids and fatty acids.

Neuron Nerve cells that exist throughout the body, but are highly concentrated in the brain, and form the 'road map' of our nervous system.

Neurotransmitter A molecule capable of stimulating a neuron. Neurotransmitters are therefore the nervous system's chemicals of communication and are usually made out of amino acids.

Phospholipid A type of semi-essential nutrient, both made by the body and required in the diet for optimal health, that is part of the membrane (myelin sheath) of neurons. Two types of phospholipids, phosphatidyl choline and phosphatidyl serine, are especially important for optimal health and brain function.

Receptor site The docking port for neurotransmitters, embedded in the membrane of a neuron. Receptor sites are specific for different kinds of neurotransmitters.

Selective Serotonin Re-uptake Inhibitor (SSRI) A type of antidepressant drug that inhibits the neurotransmitter serotonin being re-uptaken into the neuron from which it was released, hence keeping more serotonin in action.

Serotonin A neurotransmitter associated with mood, sleep patterns, dreaming and visions. It influences many physiological functions, including blood pressure, digestion, body temperature and pain sensation. Serotonin also affects mood, as well as circadian rhythm, the body's response to the cycles of day and night.

Synapse The gap between the dendrite and the neuron to which it connects. Neurotransmitters move from one neuron to another across the gap, or synapse.

Tolerance The need for increased doses of a substance over time to maintain the same effect as a result of 'downregulation'.

Upregulation The opening up of neurotransmitter receptor sites as a consequence of under-stimulation, such as withdrawal from an addictive substance, resulting in less need for external stimulants.

Withdrawal The appearance of unpleasant symptoms, which disappear when an addictive substance is reinstated.

NOTES

Chapter 2

1. GABA (gamma-amino-butyric acid), an inhibitory neurotransmitter, is associated with relaxation. It has a quietening or dampening effect on the central nervous system, and controls the release of dopamine in the reward centre of the brain. A prime example of a GABA-enhancing drug is the tranquilliser Valium. Adequate levels of GABA lead to emotional tranquillity, while low levels of GABA are associated with anxiety, tension and insomnia.

2. Adrenalin (epinephrine in the US) is associated with motivation, drive, energy, stimulation and the stress response. Produced by the adrenal glands, it is also classified as a hormone – which is a chemical messenger produced by the glands of the endocrine system. The hormonal system, while functioning at a much slower pace than the nervous system, works with the nervous system to maintain internal balance and harmony. The adrenal glands are the core of the endocrine system's stress response. They produce about 40 hormones, responsible for many body functions. Two of their most important hormones, adrenalin and cortisol, are responsible for the 'fight or flight' response that controls how we deal with stress. This is explained in detail in Chapter 6.

Without sufficient adrenalin, we are unable to meet the stresses of life. However, in response to their stressful lifestyles, most people are pumping out too much of it, causing symptoms such as: racing heart or irregular heartbeats; irritability, nervousness, anxiety, even pain; raised blood pressure; insomnia; cold hands and feet; excessive sweating; muscle tension, leading to back or neck pain, teeth grinding, headaches, even migraines; stomach pains, diarrhoea.

This 'adrenalin high' can become addictive. When the stimulus stops, such as when a stress addict goes on vacation, they actually experience adrenalin withdrawal, accompanied by restlessness, vague feelings of unease and a strong desire to 'do something', anything, to restart the stress cycle, and get the adrenalin pumping.

3. Dopamine and noradrenalin are associated with pleasure, alertness, concentration and euphoria. While both adrenalin and noradrenalin are raised by stress, noradrenalin levels tend to be higher in 'positive' stress states including sex, being 'in love', exercise, dancing or listening to music. Both dopamine and noradrenalin are made from the amino acid tyrosine and are classified as catecholamines (see the figure on pages 12–13). Dopamine appears to be the primary neurotransmitter of reward, through the dopamine receptors located in a small area of the brain called the *nucleus accumbens*. This is part of the limbic system, which governs emotions. Under stress, we release a hundred times more dopamine than we do in a normal resting state. For details, see Chapter 5, 'Stimulants'.

Adequate levels of dopamine allow one to focus to complete tasks, to feel energised and motivated and able to experience pleasure. Low levels are associated with: depression, difficulty in concentrating, difficulty in initiating and/or completing tasks and lack of motivation.

4. Endorphins is a popular term for substances known as 'opiate peptides', which include enkephalins and dynorphins. These are associated with pleasure, orgasm, euphoria and pain relief. Endorphins are the brain's own natural opiates: they bind to a specific opiate receptor, reducing pain and promoting mild euphoria, such as 'runner's high'. Interestingly, the opiates morphine and codeine are actually found in normal cerebrospinal fluid, which surrounds the brain and spinal cord.

Low levels of endorphins are associated with: physical and emotional pain, addiction and risk-taking behaviour.

5. Serotonin is associated with mood, sleep patterns, dreaming and visions. It influences many physiological functions, including blood pressure, digestion, body temperature and pain sensation. Serotonin also affects mood, as well as circadian rhythm, the body's response to the cycles of day and night.

Adequate levels of serotonin provide emotional and social stability, while low levels of serotonin are associated with: depression; anxiety; premenstrual syndrome (PMS); increased sexual drive; carbohydrate cravings; sleep disturbances; increased sensitivity to pain; emotional volatility, including violent behaviour against self and others; obsessive thinking; alcohol and drug abuse; suicide.

6. Acetylcholine is associated with memory, mental alertness, learning ability and concentration. Acetylcholine deficiency can lead to memory loss, depression, mood disorders and possibly even Alzheimer's disease. It is also the neurotransmitter at all nerve-muscle cell junctions that allows skeletal muscles to contract, controlling movement, coordination and muscle tone.

Adequate levels of acetylcholine provide mental alertness and agility while low levels of acetylcholine are associated with: poor learning; memory loss; poor concentration; difficulty visualising; lack of dreaming; dry mouth.

7. K. A. Smith et al, 'Relapse of depression after rapid depletion of tryptophan', *Lancet*, vol. 349, pp. 915–19.

Chapter 3

1. D. Benton, 'Effect of vitamin and mineral supplementation on intelligence of a sample of school children', *Lancet*, vol. 1 (23 January 1988), pp. 140–44.

2. 'Eat right and take a multivitamin', *New England Journal of Medicine* (9 April 1998), pp. 1060–61.

Chapter 4

1. M. Lader, 'Benzodiazepines – the opiate of the masses?', *Neuroscience*, vol. 3 (1978), pp. 159–65.

2. Robert Julien, *A Primer of Drug Action*, Freeman and Co. (1998), p. 340.

3. H. Woelk et al, 'Double-blind study: kava extract versus benzodiazepines in treatment of patients suffering from anxiety', *Z Allg Med*, vol. 69 (1993), pp. 271–7; D. Lindenberg et al, 'Kava in comparison with oxazepam in anxiety disorders: a double-blind study of clinical effectiveness', *Fortschr Med*, vol. 108 (1990), pp. 49–50.

4. T. F. Münte, H. J. Heinze, M. Matzke and J. Steitz, 'Effects of oxazepam and an extract of kava root (*Piper methysticum*) on event-related potentials in a word-recognition task', *Neuropsychobiology*, vol. 27, no. 1 (1993), pp. 46–53.

5. H. P. Volz and M. Kieser, 'Kava-kava extract WS 1490 versus placebo in anxiety disorders – a randomized placebo-controlled 25-week outpatient trial', *Pharmacopsychiat.*, vol. 30 (1997), pp. 1–5.

6. I. S. Shiah and N. Yatham, 'GABA functions in mood disorders: an update and critical review', *Nature Life Sciences*, vol. 63, no. 15 (1998), pp. 1289–1303.

7. Ibid.

Chapter 5

1. J. James, 'Acute and chronic effects of caffeine on performance, mood, headache and sleep', *Neuropsychobiology*, vol. 38 (1998), pp. 32–42.

2. K. Gilliland and D. Andress, 'Ad lib caffeine consumption, symptoms of caffeinism, and academic performance', *American Journal of Psychiatry*, vol. 138, no. 4 (1981), pp. 512–14.

3. J. Carper, *Your Miracle Brain*, HarperCollins (2000).

4. *Science* (11 February 2000), news report.

5. A. Astrup, 'The effect of ephedrine/caffeine mixture on energy expenditure and body composition in obese women', *Metabolism*, vol. 41, no. 7 (1992), pp. 686–8.

6. M. Blumenthal and P. King, 'Ma huang: ancient herb, modern medicine, regulatory dilemma: a review of the botany, chemistry, medicinal uses, safety concerns and legal status of ephedra and its alkaloids', *HerbalGram*, vol. 134 (1995), pp. 22–57.

7. E. Ploss, *Panax ginseng*, Kooperation Phytopharmaka, Cologne (1988), and U. Sonnenborn and Y. Proppert, 'Panax ginseng', *Z. Phytotherapie*, vol. 11 (1990), pp. 35–49. Both papers quoted in V. Schultz et al, *Rational Phytotherapy*, Springer (1998), p. 272; I. I. Brekman and I. V. Dardymov, 'New substances of plant origin which increase non-specific resistance', *Annual Review of Pharmacology and Toxicology*, vol. 9 (1969), pp. 419–30.

8. R. C. Balagot, 'Analgesia in mice and humans by D-phenylalanine: relation to inhibition of enkephalin degradation and enkephalin levels', *Advances in Pain Research and Therapy*, vol. 5 (1983), pp. 289–92; K. Budd, 'Use of D-phenylalanine, an enkephalinase inhibitor, in the treatment of intractable pain', *Advances in Pain Research and Therapy*, vol. 5 (1983), pp. 305–8.

9. H. C. Sabelli and J. Fawcett et al, 'Clinical studies on the phenylethylamine hypothesis of affective disorder', *Journal of Clinical Psychiatry*, vol. 47 (1986), pp. 66–70.

10. H. Beckmann and D. Athen et al, 'DL-phenylalanine versus imipramine: a double-blind controlled study', *Archives of Psychiatric Diseases* (*Arch Psych Nervenkr*), vol. 227 (1979), pp. 49–58.

11. J. B. Deijen et al, 'Tyrosine improves cognitive performance and reduces blood pressure in cadets', *Brain Research Bulletin*, vol. 48(2) (1999), pp. 203–9.

Chapter 6

1. P. S. Godfrey et al, 'Enhancement of recovery from psychiatric illness by methylfolate', *Lancet*, vol. 336 (1990), pp. 392–5.

2. A. Dubini et al, 'Do noradrelanin and serotonin differentially affect social motivation and behaviour?', *European Neuropsychopharmacology*, vol. 7, supplement 1 (1997), pp. S49–55.

3. K. A. Smith et al, 'Relapse of depression after rapid depletion of tryptophan', *Lancet*, vol. 349 (1997), pp. 915–19.

4. D. Eccleston, 'L-tryptophan and depressive illness', *Psychiatric Bulletin*, vol. 17 (1993), pp. 223–4.

5. K. Linde et al, 'St John's wort for depression: an overview and meta-analysis of randomised clinical trials', *British Medical Journal*, vol. 313, no. 7052 (1996), pp. 253–8.

6. E. U. Vorbach et al, 'Efficacy and tolerability of St John's wort extract LI 160 vs. imipramine in patients with severe depressive episodes according to ICD-10', *Pharmacopsychiatry*, vol. 30, supplement 2 (1997), pp. 81–5.

7. W. Poldinger et al, 'A functional-dimensional approach to depression:

serotonin deficiency and target syndrome in a comparison of 5-hydroxy-tryptophan and fluvoxamine', *Psychopathology*, vol. 24 (1991), pp. 53–81.

8. G. M. Bressa, 'S-adenosyl-methionine as antidepressant: meta-analysis of clinical studies', *Acta Neurologica Scandanavian Supplement*, vol. 154 (1994), pp. 7–14.

9. A. Miller, 'St John's wort (*Hypericum perforatum*): clinical effects on depression', *Alternative Medicine Review*, vol. 3, no. 1 (1998), pp. 18–26.

10. Godfrey, 'Enhancement of recovery from psychiatric illness by methylfolate', *Lancet*, vol. 336 (1990), pp. 392–5.

Chapter 7

1. S. Lupien, 'Longitudinal increase in cortisol during human aging, hippocampal atrophy and memory deficits', *Nature Neuroscience*, vol. 1, no. 1 (May 1998), pp. 69–73.

2. R. M. Sapolsky, 'Why stress is bad for your brain', *Science*, vol. 273, no. 5276 (1996), pp. 749–50.

3. G. Pyapali et al, 'Prenatal dietary choline supplementation', *Journal of Neurophysiology*, vol. 79, no. 4 (April 1998), pp. 1790–96; W. H. Meck et al, *Neuroreport*, vol. 8 (1997), pp. 2831–5.

4. W. Dimpfel et al, 'Source density analysis of functional topographical EEG: monitoring of cognitive drug action', *European Journal of Medical Research*, vol. 1, no. 6 (19 March 1996), pp. 283–90.

5. Cases published in W. Dean, J. Morgenthaler, S. Fowkes, *Smart Drugs 2: the next generation*, Health Freedom Publishing (1993).

6. W. Dean and J. Morgenthaler, *Smart Drugs and Nutrients*, B & J Publications (1990).

7. T. Crook et al, 'Effects of phosphatidyl serine in age-associated memory impairment', *Neurology*, vol. 41, no. 5 (1991), pp. 644–9.

8. J. R. Hibbeln, 'Fish consumption and major depression', *Lancet*, vol. 351 (1998), p. 1213.

9. A. L. Stoll et al, 'Omega-3 fatty acids in bipolar disorder', *Archives of General Psychiatry*, vol. 56 (1999), p. 407.

10. B. J. Stordy, 'Benefit of docosahexaenoic acid supplements of dark adaptation in dyslexics', *Lancet*, vol. 346 (1995), p. 385.

11. I. Hindmarch, 'Activity of ginkgo biloba extract on short-term memory', *La Presse Medicale*, vol. 15, no. 31 (1995), pp. 1562–92.

12. M. Allard, 'Treatment of old age disorders with ginkgo biloba extract', *La Presse Medicale*, vol. 15, no. 31 (1995), p. 1540.

13. E. Funfgeld, 'A natural and broad spectrum nootropic substance for treatment of SDAT – the ginkgo biloba extract', *Progress in Clinical and Biological Research*, vol. 317 (1989), pp. 1247–60.

14. J. Kleijnin and P. Knipschild, 'Ginkgo biloba', *Lancet*, vol. 340, no. 8828 (1992), pp. 1136–9.

15. P. L. Le Bars, 'A placebo-controlled, double-blind, randomised trial on an extract of Ginkgo biloba for dementia', *Journal of the American Medical Association*, vol. 278, no. 16 (1997), pp. 1327–32.

16. I. Hindmarch et al, 'Efficacy and tolerance of vinpocetine in ambulant patients suffering from mild to moderate organic psychosyndromes', *International Clinical Psychopharmacology*, vol.6, no. 1 (1991), pp. 31–43.

17. D. Benton and G. Roberts, 'Effect of vitamin and mineral supplementation on intelligence of a sample of schoolchildren', *Lancet*, vol.1 (1988), pp. 140–44.

18. W. Snowden, 'Analysis of errors and omissions in IQ tests', *Personality and Individual Differences*, vol. 22, no. 1 (1997), pp. 131–4.

19. D. Benton et al, 'The impact of long-term vitamin supplementation on cognitive functioning', *Psychopharmacology*, vol. 117 (1995), pp. 298–305.

20. S. Loriaux et al, 'The effects of nicotinic acid (niacin) and xanthinol nicotinate on human memory in different categories of age. A double-blind study', *Psychopharmacology*, vol. 87 (1985), pp. 390–95.

21. J. W. Stewart et al, 'Low B6 levels in depressed patients', *Biological Psychiatry*, vol. 141 (1982), pp. 271–2.

22. D. Pearson and S. Shaw, *Life Extension: A Practical Scientific Approach*, Warner Books (1982).

23. J. Shabert et al, *The Ultimate Nutrient – Glutamine*, Avery Publications (1994).

24. R. T. Bartus et al, 'Profound effects of combining choline and piracetam on memory enhancement and cholinergic function in aged rats', *Neurobiology of Ageing*, vol. 2 (1981), pp. 105–11.

25. S. Ferris et al, 'Combination of choline/piracetam in the treatment of senile dementia', *Psychopharmacology Bulletin*, vol. 18 (1982), pp. 94–8.

Chapter 8

1. R. Doblin et al, 'Dr Oscar Janiger's pioneering LSD research: a forty year follow-up', *Multidisciplinary Association for Psychedelic Studies Journal*, vol. 9, no. 1 (1999). Available on www.maps.org.
2. R. Dykhuizen et al, 'Ecstasy induced hepatitis', *Gut*, vol. 36 (1995), pp. 939–41; R. de Man et al, 'Acute liver failure caused by MDMA', *Nederlands Tijdschrift voor Geneeskunde*, vol. 137 (1993), pp. 727–9.
3. G. Hatzidimitriou, U. D. McCann and G. A. Ricaurte, 'Altered serotonin innervation patterns in the forebrain of monkeys treated with MDMA seven years previously: factors influencing abnormal recovery', *Journal of Neuroscience*, vol. 19, no. 12 (15 June 1999), pp. 5096–107.
4. U. D. McCann and G. A. Ricaurte et al, 'Positron emission tomographic evidence of MDMA (Ecstasy) on brain serotonin neurons in human beings', *Lancet*, vol. 352, no. 9138 (31 October 1998), p. 1437.
5. J. Marsh et al, 'Aplastic anaemia following exposure to MDMA', *British Journal of Haematology*, vol. 88 (1994), pp. 281–5.
6. McCann and Ricaurte et al, 'Positron emission tomographic evidence of MDMA (Ecstasy) on brain serotonin neurons in human beings' (1998).
7. Review available on www.erowid.org/chemicals/mdma/references/mdma_overview_memory1.shtml.
8. G. Dowling et al, ' "Eve" and "ecstasy": a report of five deaths associated with the use of MDEA and MDMA', *Journal of the American Medical Association*, vol. 257 (1987), pp. 1615–17; S. Manchanda and M. Connolly, 'Cerebral infarction in association with ecstasy abuse', *Postgraduate Medical Journal*, vol. 69 (1993), pp. 874–9; R. Harrington et al, 'Life-threatening interactions between HIV-1 protease inhibitors and the illicit drugs MDMA and gamma-hydroxybutyrate', *Archives of Internal Medicine*, vol. 159 (1999), pp. 2221–4.
9. H. Cass, 'SAMe – the master tuner supplement for the 21st century', published on www.naturallyhigh.co.uk.
10. A. Hoffer, H. Osmond et al, 'Treatment of schizophrenia with nicotinic

acid and nicotinamide', *Journal of Clinical Experimental Psychopathology*, vol. 18 (1957), pp. 131–58.

11. C. Pfeiffer et al, 'Treatment of pyroluric schizophrenia with large doses of pyridoxine and zinc', *Journal of Orthomolecular Psychiatry*, vol. 3 (1974), pp. 292–3; and C. Pfeiffer et al, 'Copper, zinc, manganese, niacin and pyridoxine in the schizophrenias', *Journal of Applied Nutrition*, vol. 27 (1975), pp. 9–39.

12. P. Godfrey at al, 'Enhancement of recovery from psychiatric illness', *Lancet*, vol. 336 (1990), pp. 392–5.

13. E. Lemert, 'Secular use of kava in Tonga', *Quarterly Journal of Studies on Alcohol*, vol. 18 (1967), pp. 328–41.

14. T. McNally in H. Cass and T. McNally, *Kava: Nature's Answer to Stress, Anxiety and Insomnia*, Prima Publishing (1998).

15. M. Smith et al, 'Psychoactive constituents of the genus sceletium: a review', *Journal of Ethnopharmacology*, vol. 50, no. 3 (1996), pp. 119–30.

Chapter 12

1. D. S. Silverberg, 'Non-pharmacological treatment of hypertension', *Journal of Hypertension Supplement*, vol. 894 (September 1990), pp. 521–6.

Chapter 13

1. M. M. Delmonte, 'Physiological concomitants of meditation practice', *International Journal of Psychosomatics*, vol. 31 (1984), p. 23.

2. J. K. Keicolt-Glaser et al, 'Modulation of cellular immunity in medical students', *Journal of Behavioural Medicine*, vol. 9 (1986), p. 5.

3. M. M. Delmonte, 'Meditation as a clinical intervention strategy: a brief review', *International Journal of Psychosomatics*, (1984), p. 31.

4. Ibid.

5. J. Thornton, *A Field Guide to the Soul: A Down-to-Earth Handbook of Spiritual Practice*, Bell Tower/Crown Publishers (1999).

6. O. Ichazo, *Interviews with Oscar Ichazo*, Arica Institute Press (1982).

Chapter 16

1. Mehmet Oz, *Healing from the Heart*, Penguin Books (1998), p. 106.

Chapter 17

1. Winnifred Cutler, 'Human sex-attractant pheromones: discovery, research, development and application in sex therapy', *Psychiatric Annals – The Journal of Continuing Psychiatric Education*, vol. 20, no. 1 (1999), pp. 54–9.

Chapter 18

1. Damien Downing, *Daylight Robbery*, Arrow Books (1988).
2. F. Lefebure, *Phosphenism*, Psychotechnic Publications (1990).
3. Downing, *Daylight Robbery* (1988), pp. 58–9.
4. M. Pathak, 'Activation of the melanocyte system by ultraviolet radiation and cell transformation', *Annals of the New York Academy of Sciences*, vol. 453 (1985), pp. 328–39.
5. L. Hinkle and H. Wolff, 'Ecologic investigation of the relationship between illness, life experiences and the social environment', *Annals of Internal Medicine*, vol. 49 (1958), pp. 1373–88.

Chapter 20

1. *Brain/Mind Bulletin* (21 January and 11 February 1985) 1–3 (out of print).

Chapter 21

1. Gallup Organization, *Sleep in America: A National Survey of US Adults*, National Sleep Foundation, Princeton (1998).
2. For details of this study, see www.nytimes.com/library/national/science/health/030700hth-sleep-memory.html.

Appendix

1. M. Lader, 'Dependence on benzodiazepines', *Journal of Clinical Psychiatry*, vol. 44 (1983), pp. 121–7.

2. Edward Drummond, *Overcoming Anxiety Without Tranquillisers*, Dutton Books (1997).

3. G. Oster et al, 'Benzodiazepines and the risk of traffic accidents', *American Journal of Public Health*, vol. 80 (1990), pp. 1467–70.

4. M. E. Tinetti et al, 'Risk factors for falls among elderly persons living in the community', *New England Journal of Medicine*, vol. 319 (1988), pp. 1701–7; and S. R. Cummings et al, 'Epidemiology of osteoporosis and osteoporotic fracture', *Epidemiologic Review*, vol. 7 (1985), pp. 178–208.

5. M. Lader, 'Benzodiazepines – the opiate of the masses?', *Neuroscience*, vol. 3 (1978), pp. 159–65.

RECOMMENDED READING

The following books will help you dig deeper into the subjects covered in this book:

General

Dr Ray Sahelian, *Mind Boosters*, St Martin's Press, 2000
Jean Carper, *Your Miracle Brain*, HarperCollins, 2000
Daniel Goldman, *Emotional Intelligence*, Bloomsbury, 1999

Chapter 3 Natural High Basics

Patrick Holford, *The Optimum Nutrition Bible*, Piatkus, 1997

Chapter 4 Relaxants

Peter Levine and Ann Frederick, *Waking the Tiger Within*, North Atlantic Books, 1997
Hyla Cass and Terrence McNally, *Kava: Nature's Answer to Stress, Anxiety and Insomnia*, Prima Publishing, 1998

Chapter 6 Mood Enhancers

Dr Hyla Cass, *St John's Wort: Nature's Blues Buster*, Avery Publishing, 1997

Chapter 7 Mind and Memory Boosters

Dr Dharma Singh Khalsa, *Brain Longevity*, Warner Books, 1999
Ward Dean MD and John Morgenthaler, *Smart Drugs and Nutrients*, Smart Publications, Santa Cruz, CA, 1990 (see www.smart-publications.com or call 707 284 3125)
Ward Dean, John Morgenthaler and Stephen Fowkes, *Smart Drugs 2: The Next Generation*, Smart Publications, Santa Cruz, CA, 1993

Chapter 8 Connectors

Richard Rudgley, *The Encyclopaedia of Psychoactive Substances*, Abacus, 1998
Aldous Huxley, *Doors of Perception*, Flamingo, 1954
Rick Strassman, *DMT – The Spirit Molecule*, Park Street Press, 1999

Chapter 10 Exercise

Gabrielle Roth, *Sweat Your Prayers, Movement as Spiritual Practice*, Penguin, 1999

Chapter 14 Biofeedback, Relaxation and the Alpha State

Herbert Benson MD, *The Relaxation Response*, Thorsons, 2000
Jim Robbins, *Symphony in the Brain: The Evolution of the New Brain Wave Biofeedback*, Atlantic Monthly Press, 2000

Chapter 15 Positive Thinking

Harville Hendrix PhD, *Getting the Love You Want*, Pocketbooks, 1993
Piero Ferrucci, *What We May Be*, J P Tarcher, 1993
Graham Stedman, *You Can Make it Happen. A 9-step Plan for Success*, NY Fireside Books, 1997

Chapter 16 The Power of Touch

Dr Mehmet Oz, *Healing from the Heart*, Penguin Books, 1998
Jaqueline Young, *Self Massage*, Thorsons, 1992

Chapter 17 Sexual Chemistry

Margo Anand, *The Art of Sexual Ecstasy*, HarperCollins, 1999
Margo Anand, *The Art of Everyday Ecstasy*, Piatkus, 1998

Chapter 20 The Music of the Emotions

Mitchell L. Gaynor MD, *Sounds of Healing: A Physician Reveals the Therapeutic Power of Sound, Voice and Music*, Broadway Books, 1999
Joshua Leeds, *The Power of Sound*, Healing Arts Press, 2001

RESOURCES

Useful Addresses

www.naturallyhigh.co.uk

Visit our website for up-to-date information on:

- The latest natural high products and suppliers
- The latest research and information on legal, natural, mind-altering substances
- Your questions answered
- Natural high seminars and events near you
- Natural high books, CDs and other resources.

The website also contains features on:

- Ecstasy – What the Research Really Shows
- Smart Drugs and Hormones – The Whole Story
- The History of Getting High
- Cannabis – The Royal Commission's Report
- SAMe and TMG – The Master Tuners
- DMT – The Spirit Molecule
- And much more.

US readers can visit us at www.highnaturally.com

Aromatherapy

Naturally High Ltd., PO Box 31729, London SW15 2GH Tel: 020 8870 9119
Produce a range of aromatherapy oils based on the research in this book. For more details visit www.naturallyhigh.shop.com or call for a catalogue.

Laboratory testing

Great Smokies' UK agent, Health Interlink, Interlink House, 1A Crown Street, Redbourn, Herts AL3 7JX. Tel: 01582 794094
Great Smokies Laboratory offer a range of tests, including those for adrenal function, DHEA levels and thyroid function. A nutritionist can arrange for you to have these tests, otherwise contact Great Smokies.

Lighting

FSL, Unit 1, Riverside Business Centre, Victoria Street, High Wycombe, Bucks HP11 2LT. Tel: 01494 448727 and Higher Nature (see Supplement Directory)
Both supply a wide range of full-spectrum lighting, including bulbs and tubes.

Massage

International Society for Professional Aromatherapists. Tel: 01455 637987
For an aromatherapy massage, call for a list of aromatherapists in your area. Also ask in your local alternative health centre.

Meditation

Siddha Yoga Meditation Centre, 32 Cubitt Street, London WC1X 0LR. Tel: 020 7278 0035

The London Buddhist Centre, 51 Roman Road, London E2 0HU. Tel: 020 8981 1225

There are countless meditation approaches and courses available. Two that have received good feedback are the one-day Learn to Meditate courses offered by Siddha Yoga and courses at the London Buddhist Centre. Both groups have regional networks.

Nutrition

Holford & Associates, 34 Wadham Road, London SW15 2LR.
For a personal referral by Patrick Holford to a clinical nutritionist in your area, visit www.patrickholford.com or write to the above address enclosing your name, address, telephone number and brief details of your health issue.

Positive thinking

There are many personal development courses available and what's right for you depends very much on your needs. Having said that here are a few powerful courses for personal transformation that we can recommend from personal experience. Also read the books recommended for Chapter 15.

The Essentials

A 2-weekend opportunity to look at how your life is, how you would like it to be and what needs to change. A great environment to look more deeply at the meaning and purpose of your life. Run by the Psychosynthesis and Education Trust (see Psychotherapy section for contact details).

The Forum

Landmark Education, 203 Eversholt Street, London NW1 1BU. Tel: 020 7969 2020.
A 3-day course providing rapid, profound transformation for living life fully.

The Hoffman Process

Hoffman Institute, The Old Post House, Burpham, Arundel BN18 9RH. Tel: 0800 0687114 or visit www.quadrinity.com
A week-long residential course that thoroughly 'undoes' negative patterns of behaviour we inherit from childhood, resulting in a profound transformation in relating and relationships and the sense of who you are.

The Quest

The Quest, PO Box 5869, Forres, Morayshire, Scotland IV36 3WG. Tel: 01309 692155 or visit www.thequest.org.uk
A home- and community-based course for exploring your own spiritual and personal development. You follow it over a period to suit yourself – from 20 weeks to a year – and go on using it for a lifetime! You can do it wherever you live, by yourself, with a partner, with a group in your community or even in a group on the Internet.

Also consider one-on-one psychotherapy or counselling (see below).

Psychocalisthenics

There are two ways to learn *Psychocalisthenics*. These are, in order of preference:

Psychocalisthenics group and individual training

MetaFitness, Squire's Hill House, Tilford, Surrey GU10 2AD. Tel: 01252 782661
This is the fastest, most effective and enjoyable way of learning the exercises in a single day. For details of training in the UK, contact MetaFitness. Expert instructors are also available to give one-to-one tuition. If you have a group of people who wish to learn *Psychocalisthenics* you can, again, arrange a teaching day with an expert instructor.

Self-tuition kit

P/CALS UK, PO Box 388, Wembley HA9 9GP. Tel: 020 8728 0211. Fax: 020 8930 7311. Email: info@pcals-uk.com. Website: www.pcals.com You can teach yourself by ordering the self-tuition kit: the book *Master Level Exercise, Psychocalisthenics* by Oscar Ichazo, a video, a wall chart and a music cassette with voice guide, cost £58, available from P/CALS UK.

Psychotherapy and Counselling

Psychosynthesis and Education Trust. Tel: 020 7403 7814
Call for a referral to your nearest/most suitable counsellor. For other information, including the Essentials courses, Tel: 020 7403 2100.

British Association for Counselling, 1 Regent Place, Rugby CV21 2PJ. Tel: 01788 550899
Contact this umbrella organisation for a list of registered counsellors in your area.

Another option is 'life coaching'. This is not therapy and life coaches do not require the same qualifications as a therapist. They act as facilitators to help you achieve your goals. For more details, and to find life coaches in your area, do a web search on 'lifecoach'.

Sound and Music

A selection of CDs listed in Chapter 20 and those of Stephen Halpern and Gabrielle Roth is available to order via the web at www.naturallyhigh.co.uk. To order by phone please call 020 8871 2949. Dr Fehmi's tapes can be ordered from www.openfocus.com. To find out about Gabrielle Roth's 5 Rhythms dance workshops and classes visit www.gabrielleroth.com.

T'ai chi

The London School of T'ai Chi Chuan and Traditional Health Resources, PO Box 9836, London SE3 0ZG. Tel: 07626 914 540 or visit www.gn.apc.org/taichi

Taoist T'ai Chi Society of Great Britain, Bounstead Road, Blackheath, Colchester, Essex CO2 0DE. Tel: 01206 576167

Also try your local alternative health centres or health-food stores for details of local classes, and check in *Yellow Pages* under sports clubs and associations, complementary therapies or martial arts or visit www.taichiunion.com.

Yoga

The British Wheel of Yoga. Tel: 01529 303233
They can put you in touch with a yoga school or teacher in your area.

Triyoga, 6 Erskine Road, Primrose Hill, London NW3 3AJ. Tel: 020 7483 3344
Offers classes all day and every day in all different types of yoga. Call for details or check out their website www.triyoga.com.

Iyengar Yoga Institute, 223a Randolph Avenue, Maida Vale, London W9 1NL. Tel: 020 7624 3080
They can put you in touch with Iyengar teachers both in the UK and around the world. Visit their website www.iyi.org.uk.

Useful Websites

www.biocybernaut.com

Dr James Hardt, director of the Biocybernaut Training Institute, describes how hundreds of people who have had profound spiritual experiences during the course of their Biocybernaut EEG training, with life-transforming results.

www.biopsychiatry.com

This website explores the subject of maximising human potential and promoting well-being through an in-depth understanding of our biochemical programming. Well worth a read. Fascinating material.

www.ceri.com

Cognitive Enhancement Research Institute (CERI) is the best way to keep up to date on mind and memory boosters. This website has many interesting features, international listings for suppliers of smart drugs and nutrients and will keep you updated on topical issues. For books on this subject also visit www.smart-publications.com.

www.heffter.org

An organisation dedicated to researching the effects of entheogens and the frontiers of neuroscience and consciousness.

www.herbalgram.org.

Ephedra Committee of AHPA, the American Herbal Products Association (www.ahpa.org) and the American Botanical Council.

www.maps.org

The website of the Multidisciplinary Association for Psychedelic Studies (MAPS) – a membership-based non-profit research and educational organisation which helps scientists to design, fund, obtain approval for and report on studies into the healing and spiritual potentials of MDMA, psychedelic drugs and marijuana. Their stated goal is 'to use the data generated from scientific research to develop these drugs into prescription medicines'.

www.rickstrassman.com

Author of *DMT – The Spirit Molecule*, psychiatrist Rick Strassman has very thoroughly researched the role of DMT with far reaching implications for understanding the association of chemistry and consciousness and the role of natural connectors.

Supplement Directory

Naturally High Ltd, PO Box 31729, London SW15 2GH.
Tel: 020 8870 9119
Produce a wide range of supplements, drinks, aromatherapy oils and other
products based on the research in this book. For more details visit
www.naturallyhigh.shop.com or call for a catalogue.

Higher Nature, Burwash Common, East Sussex, TN19 7LX.
Tel: 01435 882880. Email: sales@higher-nature.co.uk
Produce an extensive range of nutritional and herbal supplements based
on the research in this book. Available by mail order. Call for a full colour
catalogue and free newsletter.

Solgar, Solgar Vitamins Limited, Aldbury, Tring, Herts HP23 5PT.
Tel: 01442 890355
Produce a wide range of nutritional and herbal supplements including
GABA, taurine, DLPA, tyrosine, rhodiola and kava kava. Available in any
good health-food store. Contact for your nearest supplier.

Smart Drugs & Nutrients, www.uk4u.co.uk
This website sells a range of products including Deprynyl, DHEA
Hydergine, Piracetam and Nootropil to UK customers for personal use.
Also see www.ceri.com

www.naturallyhigh.co.uk. Also visit our website for up-to-date information
on the latest natural high products and suppliers.

INDEX

Note: References to figures are given as 137f and to the glossary as **288**.